Self Massage
&
40+ Fitness

Martin Morrissey

Self Massage & 40+ Fitness

Published by Northern Beaches Acupuncture and Massage, Elanora Heights, Australia.

ISBN: 978-0-9945260-0-7

Cover Design by John Reekie & Martin Morrissey.
Photography by Peter Morrissey, John Reekie, Grace Morrissey & Lachlan Morrissey.
Illustrations and cover art by Martin Morrissey.

PREFACE

The best things about Self Massage are that it feels great **and** it is good for you too. Self Massage helps your blood circulate better in your capillaries, helps the muscles contract and stretch more smoothly, and stimulates your feel-good hormones.

Over my 20-year career as a massage therapist and acupuncturist, there have been many times when a good result could have been a great one if only my client had had enough time and money to visit me a few more times.

While it is good to massage away muscular pain, it is even better to do so regularly and get the muscle and adjacent joint to operate more normally. This usually takes a few extra treatments after the pain goes away.

Giving my massage clients appropriate take-home exercises to do goes some way toward compensating for this. In my experience, though, results are even better when the client is shown Self Massage techniques they can use on themselves outside the clinic environment.

Self Massage is not a new idea – an acupuncturist showed me how to roll tennis balls along my back against the wall 30 years ago. An online search will reveal a few other Self Massage techniques too. To my knowledge, however, a comprehensive set of Self Massage methods to address muscular stiffness and pain for the whole body has not been published until this book.

I started working full time in bodywork in 1995. All was well until 2010 when I was diagnosed with polymyalgia rheumatica (PMR), a painful autoimmune cartilage and muscle condition. Over the following two and a half years, I not only greatly increased the frequency of using Self Massage on myself, I showed many of my clients how to do it too.

Because PMR affects the whole body, I needed to come up with new Self Massage techniques for my own aching parts, using myself as a guinea pig. Eventually, with the aid of massage, medication, osteopathy, chiropractic, acupuncture and Self Massage I made a complete recovery from my PMR. I also discovered that the clients who did the Self Massage I showed them were taking less time to recover from their muscle and joint problems.

These techniques work best when used properly and often, so please read all the descriptions carefully. I can honestly tell you that Self Massage has, at the time of writing this, cost me more money than it has earned for me. My clients are getting better faster and needing less treatment, in a similar way to how it helped me recover from PMR.

It is a painful truth that it gets harder to physically function as we age. How much your body's woes are strictly due to aging cannot be tested properly without participating actively and regularly in body maintenance and exercise.

Good posture is emphasized in this book too. Good posture is an ongoing continuous form of exercise that Self Massage will help you achieve.

The exercises recommended in this book will usually be safe for the 40+ population. If, however, you have specific ongoing muscle and joint disabilities, deformities, disease, trauma or scarring, it is best to consult your doctor about the suitability of the exercises and Self Massage techniques shown here.

Exercises that are potentially dangerous for the average over-40's person appear at the end of each exercise chapter. These "Risky Exercises" are best avoided.

The need for specialized health care from professionals will always be necessary, but if you practice the Self Massage and exercises in this book, you may reduce the need for professional treatment and reduce the cost of staying healthy. I am not aware of a cheaper or more accessible way of getting and staying fit.

Acknowledgements

Thank you to David Sparavec, for sharing his expert osteopathic observations and insights, and to physiotherapist Fiona Wolfenden for her advice about exercise.

Thank you to my brother Peter, daughter Grace and son Lachlan for their assistance with the photographs.

Martin Morrissey, Bach.App.Sc.Ac, DRM.

Sydney, Australia, 2016

DISCLAIMER

This book is intended as a general guide to Self Massage and exercise. **It is not intended to replace medical advice or therapy.**

If you are undergoing professional health treatment, please inform your practitioner and show them this book before you start using it, especially if you are suffering from osteoporosis or any other bone weakening condition. If you have had surgery, ask your surgeon if and when massage can be applied near or over any operated zone.

Please follow the instructions carefully. Do not attempt the more advanced exercises and Self Massage techniques until you have tried the more gentle methods.

If any activity in this book causes you pain, nausea, dizziness or breathlessness, stop that activity immediately. If the symptoms persist, seek medical attention.

Please be sure to read the **Safety First** chapter before attempting any activity in this book.

FURTHER INFORMATION

At my website, martinmorrissey.net, you can find further information about issues affecting your muscle and joint health. The effects of occupation, eating habits, environment, stress, attitude and seemingly unrelated health conditions can have some surprising influences on our musculoskeletal health.

You will also find definitions, suggested treatments, self-help information and preventative strategies for some of the more common muscular and rheumatic diseases. The articles are easy to follow, approximately 1 page each (500 words), and frequently updated and indexed for easy location.

You can find also answers to commonly asked questions and leave your own queries and comments.

http://martinmorrissey.net/

TABLE OF CONTENTS

PART I

Introduction and explanations of Self Massage and exercise.

PART II

Self Massage and exercises for all areas of your body.

PART III

Advanced techniques and branching out.

PART IV

Introductory programs for different activities. Golf, a popular 40+ activity, gets its own chapter.

PART I

Introduction and explanations of Self Massage and exercise.

1 INTRODUCTION

Life rarely gets simpler. There is always something more to fit into an already crowded existence. It is hard making time for yourself when you are working so hard to keep everybody else happy.

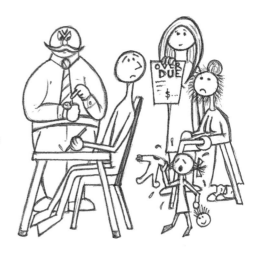

The bottom line, however, is that if you don't look after yourself, you are of no use to anybody else. Waiting too long to do something about your aches and pains may make you regret acting too late.

When we do make the time to do some exercise, accumulated muscular stiffness can make the activity uncomfortable and unproductive. By using Self Massage, you can make your body more comfortable to exercise, work and play.

What I propose in this book is to take a dual approach to wellness: Self Massage and exercise combining synergistically. We need look no further than professional sports to see how exercise and massage synergize with one another. Therapeutic massage helps keep highly paid athletes on the field by assisting with muscular recovery from injuries sustained in training and competition. The bodies of professional athletes are made of the same stuff as the rest of us.

The big common denominator between exercise and massage is that they are both great circulatory aids. Good circulation is essential to health and fitness.

In this book, I explain a series of Self Massage techniques that are easy to do – you do not need to have strong hands for them. This is made possible by utilizing simple leverage and your hands, elbows, and inexpensive massage tools.

I will also show you exercises that are most suited to the needs of the 40+ body. I will explain how to weed out common exercise practices that are unlikely to produce good results and might even cause you harm.

While this book is ostensibly written for the over-40's, the Self Massage and exercise practices recommended here can also be of benefit to people under 40. From 40 onward, however, bodies injure more easily and recover more slowly. When you look around the fitness industry, it caters mainly for those under 40. What I have set out to present in this book is something of practical value to those in the second half of their lives.

1.1 WHY SELF MASSAGE?

Massage has been around for a long time and all cultures have their own forms of hands-on healing. What is different about this book is that I will show you how to do it for yourself.

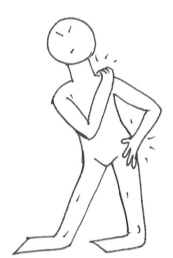

Your skeleton gives your body structure and your muscles are the motors that move your bones. Muscle accounts, on average, for 40% of body mass. Muscles lose their elasticity, strength and endurance over time; because of injury, fatigue, lack of exercise, the wrong exercises, toxin build-up, chronic dehydration, smoking, poor nutrition, bad posture, stress, overwork, disease and aging.

Your muscles are full of blood vessels. Anatomy and physiology textbooks classify the circulatory system as a transportation system, and the circulation of blood and other body fluids is central to our health and fitness. The main purpose of massage and Self Massage is to help return muscle to its normal relaxed state by assisting the blood circulation in the muscles at a capillary level. They promote smoother muscle function by assisting the pumping of blood through the muscle tissue, removing waste products, freeing up trauma adhesions and assisting transport of oxygen and nutrients to your extremities.

Massage also helps us by stimulating "feel-good" hormones like dopamine, serotonin and oxytocin. You can feel uplifted for hours by the actions of these hormones. Massage provides stress relief as well as physical ease. Stress hormones like cortisol and noradrenaline are suppressed by massage too.

Self Massage helps you to do this for yourself for no cost other than what you have spent on this book and a few cheap massage tools. It can be done in the comfort of your own home while you are watching TV or listening to the radio. It is that simple – you just need to follow the instructions. You do not need strong hands to do the majority of the Self Massage techniques. It's all about positioning your body correctly and applying pressure in the right direction with the right tools.

Even so, if you have never had a professional massage before, I recommend that you get one. It will help you know how a good massage should feel. Even if you don't think that you need it, you should try it, as it is easy to forget what it is like to feel normal. When you attempt Self Massage, try to make yourself feel the same way.

1.2 WHY EXERCISE?

Whether you are male or female, old or young, exercising the right way will make you look better and help you feel good. There is no product that you can buy that can take the place of exercise, and nobody can do it for you.

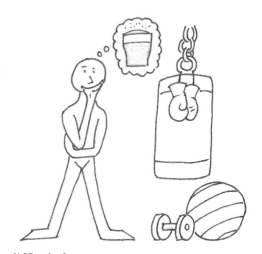

Exercise improves muscular strength, flexibility, endurance and coordination. It lowers blood pressure, makes you more sure-footed, mentally sharpens you, and helps you feel warm when it is cold outside.

Exercise strengthens your bones and helps protect you from diabetes. The hormones it releases into your bloodstream can raise your spirits even if life is difficult for you.

Exercise tells that lover that just dumped you, "So what, I can find someone else." It helps us reinvent ourselves and can be very cathartic. Parents and grandparents who exercise are more likely to have kids and grandkids who will exercise. Exercising with them can bring you closer to them, teaching them self-respect and confidence and making them feel proud of you.

Exercise can be the difference between recovering from a major injury and giving into addiction and losing hope – something I saw too often when I was a nurse. A growing number of medical practitioners are recommending exercise to patients who are suffering from depression. We are learning new things all the time about how exercise helps us.

By the time we are 40, we really have to think about how we are going to be at retirement age and beyond. I have been fortunate enough to have met people who have been fit, lithe, energetic and mentally sharp well into their 80's. They are inspiring – living proof of what is possible. They also started doing something about it much earlier on.

Most of the things that go wrong with us are not due to our DNA. Rather, it is because of the choices we make. Making good choices buys us time and peace of mind. Vanity may not be the noblest motivation to exercise but if that's what it takes to get fit and stay that way, so be it. Who doesn't want to look good?

As we age, the exercise that suits us best may change but that doesn't have to be a negative – change is natural and can keep life interesting. Exercise helps with digestion, sleep, stress management, breathing, blood circulation and your energy levels. It's not just about making your muscles look and feel better.

1.3   GETTING FITNESS-READY

The most important pre-requisite to improving your fitness is the will to do it, followed closely by the ability to do so.

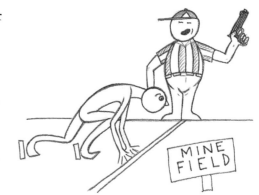

Pain and awkwardness of movement when exercising can be a big fitness obstacle for the over-40's – this is why I am promoting Self Massage as a fitness aid. Self Massage will help prepare your muscles for exercise and can be used to sooth them afterward.

Note that it may still be necessary to get some treatment for your knees, lower back, shoulders and feet from a health professional before you get into your new training. Self Massage cannot fix everything.

It is important to adopt the right attitude from the start. You should plan to exercise or do a series of Self Massage techniques **before** you do other things, not **after**. This does not mean you should train only in the morning; it means you will get better results by making a priority of it.

Your welfare – both physically and emotionally – is every bit as important as the welfare of those you take care of. If you lose sight of your own needs, your capabilities as a caregiver will diminish. If you feel you do not have the time to do healthy things, first cut back on the time you spend doing unhealthy things.

Be resourceful and adaptable about planning exercise time. For example, it is easy to stretch your neck and calves while on the train on your way to work. Take the stairs rather than the elevator if you can. Taking deep breathes and holding them in for as long as you can, several times a day, can help your lung capacity.

Many of the stretches and Self Massage techniques in this book can be done while sitting at a computer. Set an alarm on the computer to give yourself a short break every hour and do some Self Massage and stretching. Set aside a short period in the morning and the evening to work through some of the techniques that can't be done while sitting.

Getting started does not have to be expensive – the main purpose of this book is to help you improve your fitness cheaply. But don't skimp on the gear that you really do need. (For example, if you intend on road running, get good shoes for it.)

1.4 CHOOSING AN INSTRUCTOR

For some of the exercises in this book, you may feel more comfortable doing or learning them under qualified supervision, whether it be stretching, functional fitness, cardio, or strength training. Tuition from someone about the same age as yourself should give them a better insight into your needs – all other things being equal. Even better still, if they have suffered similar physical problems as yourself in the past, their insights may be of great value to you.

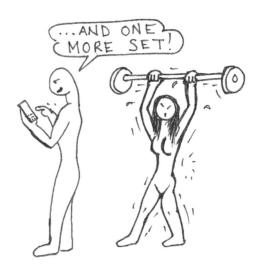

Don't be over-ambitious. If you are a beginner, go to a beginners' class. If you were fit 10 years ago but are not now, do not try to immediately attempt to pick up from where you left off.

If you cannot find a suitable beginner's class, you can choose to participate in an exercise class with others of mixed fitness levels. Ask the teacher beforehand to give you another activity to keep busy with when you cannot keep up or the activities are too hard. You can re-join in what everyone else is doing later in the class.

One-on-one tuition will cost you more, but you will learn faster and should get results quicker. Doing your tuition at home will also help you to avoid the trap of thinking that you can only exercise if you go somewhere special to do it.

A good instructor will ask relevant questions about your medical history: back pain, abnormal blood pressure, vertigo, ankles that easily twist, heart conditions, and so on. Good instructors also have the courtesy and professionalism to pay attention to what you are paying them for. If you find yourself getting bored or if you don't understand the exercise, let your instructor know. Accidents are less likely if you are mentally engaged in what you are doing.

Always remember that you are the one paying the money, so you are entitled to know what you are paying for and to receive it. There are no dumb questions, just dumb answers. If you get unconvincing or patronizing responses to your enquiries, find another instructor.

Finally, if you ever hurt yourself, **stop**. Nobody will give you a medal for pushing on through pain, whether in a class or in one-on-one training. Remember that pride comes before a fall: don't try to impress anyone, and listen to your body. Not every workout has to be a "personal best."

1.5 STAYING MOTIVATED

Weight loss is often a strong incentive for improving fitness, but it should not be the only one. Exercise provides many, many more benefits than weight loss alone.

There are many factors that may conspire to dent your motivation. It is important to notice and understand these if you want to keep improving your fitness. Be realistic with your goals and remember that it is impossible to turn back the clock. It is much more helpful to picture yourself as a fitter and slightly older you than as a younger person again.

Think about what you want to achieve and enjoy with the rest of your life. How likely are these things to happen on your current course? Health and fitness is usually something that you **earn**. Even if your genes are good, how you treat yourself is a more reliable predictor of how you will age. Change is normal, so embrace it.

Fatigue and weakness can be a huge disincentive to exercise. Your thyroid may be sluggish, testosterone low or you may be anemic. These problems are all testable and treatable, so get to the bottom of it if you want to enjoy better health and vitality.

Educate yourself about how your body works. You don't have to go to university to do this. It is easier to initiate healthy change if you can see why you should. This book is a good start.

Motivation can be undermined by social factors. As the saying goes, "It is hard to soar like an eagle when you are surrounded by turkeys." Be aware of peer influences, and seek out others that share similar goals to you. If your partner starts to get jealous or feel insecure about your new activities, encourage them to get fit with you. There is nothing wrong with wanting to look good – self-esteem is good for your confidence and health.

If you are finding an exercise program tough going, remember to balance it with stretching and Self Massage. Self Massage helps motivate you to exercise because it makes physical activity more comfortable. Muscles both stretch and flex with greater ease and reliability when massaged regularly.

"Discontent is the first necessity of progress" (Thomas Edison). We all need something to strive for. There is nothing more important in life than for you and those you love to be healthy, so make it a mission. But listen to your body and read the **Safety First** chapter. Injury is very bad for your motivation.

2   SELF MASSAGE & ITS TOOLS

In Parts II and III of this book, I will present Self Massage techniques for all areas of your body. The techniques are normally safe to do but if any of them cause pain, nausea or dizziness, please desist. If you have any doubts about the safety of any Self Massage technique, please bring this book to your favorite therapist and ask his or her opinion about what you intend on doing.

2.1   HOW TO SELF MASSAGE

The way you position your body when Self Massaging is critical, so please follow the directions for each and every technique or it won't work properly. You must feel balanced and have control over the pressure you are using at all times.

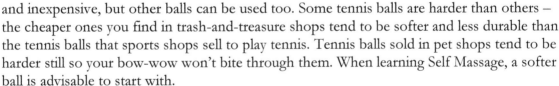

The correct pressure should feel dull, not sharp. If you feel like you are barely able to relax into the pressure, you are either going too hard or the angle you are working at is not as instructions and images demonstrate.

Many of the Self Massage techniques in this book are demonstrated with tennis balls because they are commonplace and inexpensive, but other balls can be used too. Some tennis balls are harder than others – the cheaper ones you find in trash-and-treasure shops tend to be softer and less durable than the tennis balls that sports shops sell to play tennis. Tennis balls sold in pet shops tend to be harder still so your bow-wow won't bite through them. When learning Self Massage, a softer ball is advisable to start with.

The standing techniques in this book should be done against solid walls. If you are a large person, be careful about leaning firmly against a plasterboard wall. Walls with a glossy surface are too easy for balls to slip against, so use walls with a flat (matt) non-slip surface and ensure you are standing on a non-slip surface – not in your socks on a polished floor. Stand with your feet at least a shoulder's width apart.

Do Self Massage in front of a mirror to check your body is in the right position (refer to the diagrams or photographs). Getting into the right posture is important. Some of the postures required to Self Massage can look a little odd, comical or even suggestive so you may prefer to do them in private, at least to begin with.

Be resourceful and opportunistic with using your time. You do not need a gym or a clinic to do Self Massage. You can do it while you are watching TV or waiting for files to upload or download while working at the computer.

Whenever using stroking or rolling techniques on your arms and legs, always endeavor to do so with greater pressure working upward toward your torso, to aid circulation. The more you practice, the better the results.

Please try the easier techniques before you try the harder ones. If you cannot relax into the pressure of tennis balls behind your back leaning into a wall, lying on the floor with them under you will be way too much pressure. Please thoroughly read the SAFETY FIRST chapter before starting.

The techniques in the Advanced Self Massage chapter are strongest and should be used only after getting used to the softer techniques.

2.2   SELF MASSAGE AND AGING

Sometimes after a serious injury or joint replacement surgery, people become overly cautious about exercise and massage. If you have had major surgery, ask your doctor if it is safe to exercise and get massaged. If he or she says it is OK, that is what you should do. The reason we have surgery is so we can live more fully and normally, and this book will help you to do that.

Another more common reason for people of advancing years to give up on their fitness is joint pain. Even if you have been diagnosed with arthritis, it does not mean there is nothing you can do to help yourself.

There have been numerous times over the last 20 years that clients have told me they have given up on exercise because it hurts too much. Someone may have come for a neck rub and when I ask if they are sore anywhere else, they might say "my lower back is always a bit sore but it has been like that for years, I just live with it." Maybe you don't have to live with it. Don't wait for a little pain to become a big one.

Self Massage is something you can do regularly because it costs nothing and you can do it at home. The Self Massage techniques in Parts II and III can help you rediscover lost vigor. Even if you think your legs or arms are fine just how they are, try Self Massaging them and you may find they have sensitive stiff spots you were not even aware of. After you Self Massage these areas, physical activity can become easier and more productive.

If you have had past muscle and joint trauma, you may never feel completely normal again, but it costs nothing to try Self Massage – it could help give you a new lease on life.

2.3   SELF MASSAGE AND SLEEP

My clients often fall asleep as I massage them. Neck and upper back massage in particular can help induce sleep. If you suffer from insomnia, you may be able to help yourself sleep better by Self Massaging before you go to bed.

Try some of the neck and upper back techniques and you may be surprised how much faster you can fall asleep. You are likely to wake up feeling more refreshed going to sleep this way than knocking yourself out with drugs or alcohol. Self Massage produces no side-effects either, such as night sweats or snoring.

The best way to use Self Massage to help you sleep is to do it just before you go to bed. Then as soon as you start to feel drowsy, turn in for the night. Massage raises serotonin levels in your bloodstream, which is an important precursor for melatonin, a sleep-inducing hormone.

Stress is a big contributor to insomnia. Massage activates the parasympathetic nervous system, which calms us down when we are stressed. Poor sleep is bad for your immunity, circulation and mood; it also affects your powers of concentration.

Tossing and turning to get to sleep can upset your partner's sleep too. Both of you can benefit by you Self Massaging. It is such a simple, free and easy way to promote better sleep.

2.4   THE TOOLS

Some of the Self Massage techniques are performed with your own hands and elbows. Other techniques utilize massage tools, both purpose-made and improvised. Please use the purpose-made tools according to manufacturers' instructions.

Improvised tools such as the balls, walking stick and sink plunger should only be used as demonstrated and only if they are in new or as-new condition.

When using any of these tools for the first time, always go easy. Slowly ease into full contact pressure and do not use any rocking or abrupt force. Always make sure that you feel well-balanced and in full control of the pressure.

A few of the techniques utilize wall angles and doorways. Avoid glossy slippery surfaces and please beware of the risk of someone running into you if they do not expect you to be there.

Electrical massage appliances can be useful and range from hand-held battery operated gadgets right up to heated massage tables with oscillating vibrating heads costing thousands of dollars. These appliances are not used in this book because I want to show you the cheapest, simplest and most portable Self Massage options.

Balls are versatile Self Massage tools. Tennis balls are used extensively in this book. Golf balls, squash balls, baseballs or purpose made massage balls can also be used. Use softer balls before you try using harder ones. You may find even the softer tennis balls a bit challenging when doing it for the first time, so please try the standing techniques (leaning against a wall) before attempting an advanced technique on the floor. If you have trouble getting down onto the floor, the harder balls can be more useful if you want to lie on your bed to Self Massage.

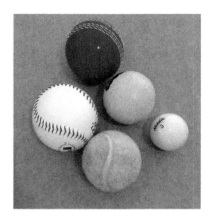

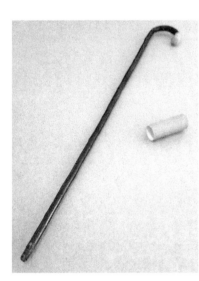

The **walking stick** is a versatile Self Massage tool. You can either apply direct contact to pressure points with the end of the handle or use the shaft to roll along your stiff muscles.

The walking stick shown at left has the end of its handle taped for greater comfort of use, but if your stick has a round smooth end it may be fine how it is.

The cardboard tube (toilet roll) acts as a rolling sleeve around the shaft of the walking stick, which makes Self Massaging your legs more comfortable. A similarly sized tube like electrical conduit is suitable too.

Don't use a weak or broken walking stick. And don't use umbrella handles, as they are not strong enough.

Massage tools of the type shown at right are common and appear in many variations. They can be purchased inexpensively online. Keep your wrist straight as you make contact with the muscles and pressure points. The rounded handle ends are useful for Self Massage of the chest and thigh muscles and the black capped stem is great for the calf muscles. It is lightweight, versatile and durable if used properly. While made for use on others, they are even more suitable for Self Massage.

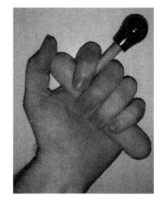

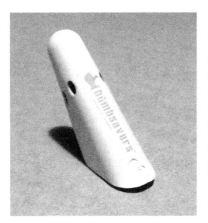

This is a **Thumbsaver**. It acts as an exoskeleton for your thumb or fingers, allowing you to exert firmer and more sustained pressure on the smaller muscles, such as in your neck, jaws, hands and feet. They are inexpensive, available online and come in different sizes to suit thumbs of different lengths. It is important for massage therapists and Self Massagers to not overuse their thumbs. Thumbsavers easily fit in your pocket, are semi-rigid and easy to use. This particular one has been used for hundreds of massages so far. While designed for use on others, I find them even more effective for Self Massage.

Foam rollers are a popular physiotherapist's tool. This one was purchased at an online physiotherapy supplies website, but you can find much cheaper identical rollers in department stores now. They can be used on your upper back, thighs and lats. Foam rollers are used to stretch and massage the muscles simultaneously. They are easy to use but can feel a bit firm when you first try, so go gently to start with.

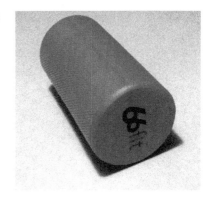

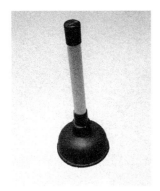

The **sink plunger** is a good tool for focused pressure. Buy a new one to try the techniques that use it in this book. It gives a good deep tissue effect for the larger muscles. For this reason it is recommended for the advanced techniques after you try the softer methods first. Always hold the shaft when you are using it, even though its suction cup can make good firm contact on the wall. You can apply cloth tape to the handle if you find the end a bit sharp.

2.5 MOODS, MUSCLES & MASSAGE

Massage and exercise can help lift your mood and confidence through raising the levels of "feel good" hormones like serotonin and dopamine. Stress, on the other hand, raises the levels of hormones like cortisol and adrenaline that do not make us feel relaxed at all.

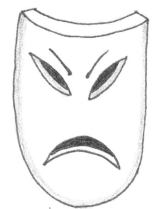

This is reflected in our muscles too. All other things being equal, you are likely to feel far more unpleasant muscular tension immediately after an emotional upset than you felt just before it. This is an instant example of how what we think can produce a noticeable and rapid muscle tension change.

During prolonged stress, our muscles can achieve a chronic tension that stiffens and weakens them. This often goes completely unnoticed – when we are stressed, it is very difficult to think about anything other than what is stressing us. (Prolonged stress weakens physical immunity too.)

This process is recognized in Chinese medicine, bio-energetics, Rolfing, Alexander technique, kinesiology and Feldenkrais. You don't need to know anything about body language at all to tell if someone is stressed – it affects our whole demeanor. You can make a heroic effort to control your reactions to something you don't like, but your muscles will still reactively stiffen. When we are apprehensive, our bodies become more rigid.

When we describe someone as a pain in the neck, our feelings about them can literally do just that to us. In acupuncture, anger is a well-known cause of painful neck muscle tension, especially when anger stays unresolved.

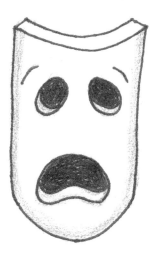

Stress can also cause muscular tension in other parts of the body. I once saw a university student rub at his tight forearms vigorously just before he was caught cheating in an exam. I only learned later on that this is a well-known physical reaction observed in people doing sneaky things.

Burglars reputedly defecate at the scene of their crimes because of the effect of high adrenaline levels on their bowel muscles. The fear of getting caught by police or security can greatly raise adrenaline levels. Everyone knows how twitchy our arm muscles get when someone really offends us. The frown that is on your face while this is happening is the result of facial muscles being stimulated by emotion too.

Adrenaline and noradrenaline have a powerful effect in priming our bodies for "flight or fight," by sending blood to our arm and leg muscles to ready them for action. These same hormones can create a muscular rigidity in our limbs that can produce a statue-like stillness, as when we are paralyzed with fear. Staying still and unnoticed sometimes can be our best form of protection. Adrenaline is there to help us survive danger.

Jaw tension is a very common stress reaction to anxiety and anger. This too is unconscious. Nobody *deliberately* gets jaw tension and the strong headaches that often go with it – it happens as a reaction to emotional excitation.

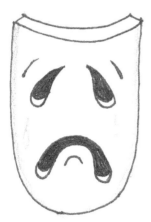

Body language is a commonplace psychosomatic reaction that demonstrates the relationship between stress and muscle action. When someone is calm and relaxed, their body language is totally different.

It probably won't be the first thing you think about when you are really upset, but doing some Self Massage and exercise can actually help raise happy hormone levels and lower the unhappy ones. There have been many times I have used Self Massage and exercise to help myself at the end of an unpleasant day.

Tiredness produces stress hormones when we push ourselves to stay awake and keep going. When we get to that point, we are more likely to make irrational decisions. Hormonal effects can really rattle us.

In over 20 years of clinical practice I have seen a number of clients who were suffering from PTSD (post traumatic stress disorder). They did not come to me for counseling, just to do something about their stiff and sore muscles.

Some of the stories I have heard from these clients were truly horrifying, and sometimes they were very emotional too. I can honestly say though that massage did seem to help them feel better. The beauty of Self Massage is you can have it every day.

When you are stressed, you are totally trapped inside your own head, but its effects do not remain confined to your head. Self Massage and exercise can help you manage your stress by attacking it from a different angle. It is empowering.

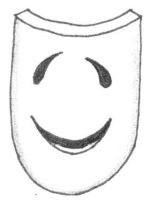

> **Self Massage and exercise are not a substitute for psychotherapy or psychiatry. Do not change your medications without a medical consultation.**

3 POSTURE

Posture is the position the body is held in when standing, sitting or lying. It is important because it affects our balance and movement. Good posture is healthy because our muscles, bones, joints and internal organs operate best when we observe it.

These illustrations are examples of what good posture looks like: your head should be held directly above the pelvis, with your chin in and shoulders back. When viewed from the side, your spine has curves in it that support your body weight best when your hips and shoulders are vertically aligned with one another. This is what defines a straight back.

Your normal standing posture should be with your feet about a shoulder's width apart, with a straight back and your head held high. When you are sitting or standing, your body works, feels and looks best when your spine is perpendicular to the ground.

A straight posture also requires equal muscle tone between the right and left sides of your body. This is why you should endeavor to have even muscular strength either side of your spine and pelvis. Your spine is strongest when held this way and is less subject to wear and tear.

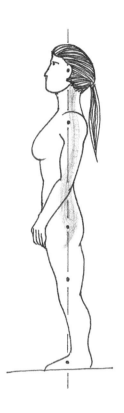

If you have bad posture (and we all fail in this department at times), it may feel "normal" because you get used to it. Like all other bad habits, bad posture can be difficult to break.

Think about a Bonsai plant and how a wire can be wrapped around it so that it will grow into a particular shape. Your postural decisions are like an invisible wire that determines the shape of your spine and other bones.

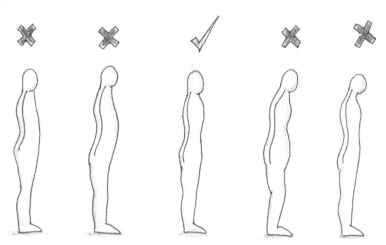

3.1 BONES AND POSTURE

It has surprised me over the years how many people I have met who don't even know they have poor posture, because it is a bad habit they have gotten used to. If we could only see what bad posture looks like on the inside, we would be more attentive to how we sit and stand.

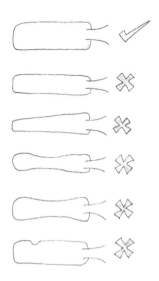

The top drawing on the right is a profile of a normal, healthy vertebra (backbone). The others are misshapen backbones that often are caused by chronic bad postural habits. Slouching can eventually change the shape of your bones and prematurely wear your discs out.

Osteopaths and chiropractors refer to spinal misalignments as *subluxations*. Injuries can cause subluxations and can result from postural faults that create weaknesses of the spine. Poor posture can distort vertebrae shape.

Sometimes postural distortions are caused by the way body weight is distributed. Often pregnant women will get lower back pain because of how their bellies pull the lower spine forward.

Overweight men are subject to this too, because they are more likely to carry excess bodyweight in the abdomen.

Tiredness, low self-esteem, stress, posture-unfriendly work, weakness and muscular stiffness all affect your posture through uneven stresses placed on your discs and vertebrae. Bad posture can be started off by many things: a leg injury or surgery that permanently changes the way you walk, an untreated hernia or poor footwear. It could just be that you unconsciously copied the way your parents moved, stood and sat.

Good posture requires effort. If you are physically lazy by nature, you will have to try extra hard to replace your bad postural habits with good ones.

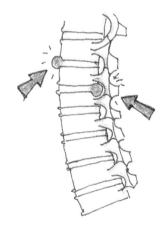

By analogy, consider a stack of children's building blocks. As you stack them to make a tower they will start to lean. Then you have to place the next block in the opposite direction so it will be straighter. Similarly, our spinal muscles have to work extra hard to correct bad posture. Spinal misalignment is hard work, and a crooked spine is more likely to get disc problems.

Illustrated at the right are pristine vertebrae and discs. The bone is smooth and the disc cartilage has maximum flexibility and cushioning from shock. This is how it looks when we are young and agile. We are at our tallest in that interval of time between our bones ceasing to grow and our discs starting to lose their thickness.

When the discs start to lose their thickness, the flexibility and shock absorption of the spine begins to noticeably diminish. When the discs get to this stage, we start to become more aware of the need to stretch. Stretching exercises help preserve the discs by assisting with blood circulation in the disc.

Chronic poor posture can change bone shape and restrict normal movement. At right, the disc has shrunk to a degree where your height noticeably lessens. Healing takes longer and greater care is needed to avoid and manage injury. When the disc deteriorates to this point, you will be aware that you cannot bend and twist your spine like you used to.

If your spine gets to the stage illustrated at right, movement is greatly restricted to the point where some joints won't move at all and posture becomes noticeably distorted. How you treat your body determines in a large part whether this happens. This cartilage is severely dehydrated and atrophied. Your vertebrae can fuse together at this stage, and even passive stretching won't move it.

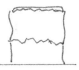

A straight spine actually curves toward the front at your neck and mid section, and toward the back at your upper back and sacrum. When viewed from the front or back, the spine should be gun-barrel straight.

While you are still reasonably young, you can make a conscious decision to start standing and sitting straight and so prevent lipping and wedging of the vertebrae. Once your bones start growing this way, it is very difficult to get them growing straight again.

Age 40 is about as late as you can leave it to sort your posture out. The next time you see an elderly person struggling at their walking frame almost bent at a right angle, consider that they were probably not born that way. They probably got there through long-term uncorrected and worsening posture that helped bring about osteoporosis, which finally reached a point where their spine started disintegrating.

The more you keep good posture, the greater the likelihood your discs will wear evenly and the less you will seem to shrink.

3.2   POSTURE AND MINDSET

Teaching kids about posture early on is a great idea – you can save them a lot of suffering later on. Kids who do ballet, gymnastics or physical culture benefit from greater postural awareness. Curiously enough though, despite girls participating in these things more often, they get deviated spines (scoliosis) much more frequently than boys do, for reasons that are not entirely clear.

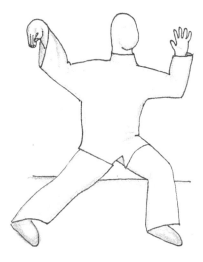

Young women do tend to be proportionately over-represented with corrective spinal surgery. Some of the reasons may be psychological. Girls who are unusually tall and/or large-breasted do tend to stoop and hold their shoulders forward in order to feel less conspicuous, particularly around boys.

If you have a daughter or granddaughter who does this, you need to intervene – if slouching becomes a habit, it is not something she will necessarily grow out of. As mentioned previously, posture can change the shape of bones. It is much easier sorting these things out early than correcting them later on. Examine your own posture too with a critical eye, because kids often mirror parental examples.

Posture and body language are closely related to one another. Even if you claim to have no specific knowledge of body language, it is nevertheless easy to make casual and correct observations about it when you see it. Women in particular are good at recognizing and using it, some say up to six times better than men.

I had the following story related to me by one of my clients years ago. B was a bus driver, and was sent by his employer with lots of other bus drivers to a self-defense in-service workshop. To B's relief, very little of the instruction involved hand-to-hand combat training; the emphasis was on diverting situations before they got out of hand.

One of the first things B and his colleagues were shown during their workshop was a series of CCTV films of muggings and bag snatchings in different public places.

Some of the victims were older, some younger, and males and females seemed equally represented amongst the victims.

The lights were then turned on and B and cohort were asked what all the victims had in common. None could answer the question accurately. So then the film was played again with the instructor talking them through it this time.

During the film the muggers could be seen letting others walk past unharrassed before a victim was chosen. What all the victims had in common was that they all looked like they wouldn't fight back, because they had the posture of someone lacking confidence.

Once this was pointed out, B could see that they were right. Even though some of the victims may have been physically larger than those allowed past, they had timid body language with crumpled postures. They did indeed look like victims before they became victims, and none fought back.

The moral of the story seems to be that if you don't have good posture naturally, it may serve you well to fake it convincingly. When you watch movies, notice how the high status characters usually stand tall, and submissive characters seem to be almost trying to hide themselves with their postures.

Frederick Alexander, an Australian actor, noticed the physical cause and effect behind posture through playing different roles and exploring how they made him feel. So much so that he developed the Alexander Technique, an interesting and useful postural health training method.

Good posture not only makes people more attractive and helps make them physically fitter, it is also a form of communication. There are many other good reasons to have good posture, even if just to avoid having unpleasant spinal surgery later on. Sometimes the surgery works well and sometimes not so much – if your posture doesn't change, for instance, optimal results are unlikely. Prevention is way cheaper than surgery too.

This is why I always insist on good posture in myself and others. I have nursed people who have slouched their way into hospital beds through years of poor posture. It really isn't worth it. I saw it happen to my own mother too – it was no fun for her at all.

If you cannot physically train yourself to better posture, you may need extra help with this. The older you get, the greater the consequences of poor posture.

3.3   POSTURE AND SITTING

The best posture for standing, sitting or even lying is one that maintains the natural curves in your spinal column. The key to achieving the healthiest posture for your back has as much to do with your legs as it does your spine.

135°

The spine is naturally segmented in such a way that if one spinal curve is changed, the others change too. This is because your head needs upright support to keep your eyes level and pointed ahead. Sitting the wrong way is bad for your whole spine, not just your lower back.

When you sit with your knees more-or-less level with your hips (as with conventional seating), it instantly flattens the normal curve of your lower back. This pushes your upper back forward, which makes the muscles behind your neck work harder than they should.

This is not a new discovery – orthopedic surgeon and researcher J.J. Keegan arrived at the conclusion in 1955 that the best way to sit is to open your hip to a 135-degree angle, not 90–100 degrees as with most chairs.

Even though saddle chairs are a relatively new invention, they are based on a much older design idea still – saddles for horses, hence the name. Unfortunately, saddle chairs are too tall to use at a desk of average height. This is a shame because we may all have better backs if they could be used. A 135-degree angle between thigh and spine gives you the strongest and most sustainable support for your lower back.

3.4   POSTURE AND DRIVING

Men tend to have different driving styles to women. One of the most obvious is the way they sit in the driver's seat, perhaps in admiration of Formula One and Indy Car drivers.

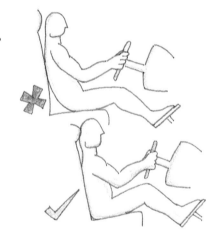

Women, on the other hand, almost always sit more bolt upright with their butt pulled right back into the seat against the backrest. This way of sitting in a car is way more posture-friendly to the lower back.

It is OK for racing drivers to be almost lying flat in their cars because that is how their seats are designed in order to accommodate the low center of gravity for high-speed cornering.

For the rest of us, the seat needs to be close enough to the dash to easily reach the pedals properly, with your butt pulled right back into the seat as far as it can go. Otherwise, it will diminish the natural curve and strength of your spine.

Gentlemen, it is time to pull that seat forward to a point where you can reach the firewall flat-footed, while keeping your butt as far back into the seat as it can go. Don't forget to adjust the mirrors when you do this.

3.5   POSTURE AND SLEEP

It is a fact that you are a full 2 cm taller first thing in the morning than you are last thing at night. This is because your vertebrae (backbones) relax apart from each other during sleep, relieving pressure on your spinal discs.

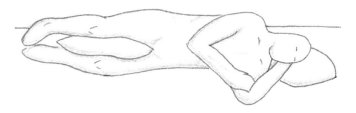

Sleeping flat on your back with a good supporting mattress is considered ideal. If you must sleep on your side, place a reasonably thick pillow between your knees, as this will help keep your spine straight. If you sleep alternating from side to back, you should use two different pillows to support your head.

If you would rather sleep supine (on your back) but don't because it makes you snore, then getting fit, losing weight, drinking less alcohol and using the reflexology technique **R1 Finger roll** (page 177) may give you and your partner a better night's sleep.

If you get sore feet, placing a pillow beneath your calves can slightly raise your heels and can make sleeping on your back easier.

Women often like lying face down. This posture is no good at all for your spine and you are more likely to inhale fabric fibers and dust mites from your sheets doing this.

All mattresses need to be rotated periodically in order to give you a flat, firm sleeping surface. Even the highest quality mattresses will eventually need replacing. Pillows wear out too. Saggy old pillows and mattresses cannot support good sleeping posture. Your spine would be better off if you slept on the floor.

Note that thick pillows can push your head too far forward. Ideally the inward curve (lordosis) of your neck needs support, particularly when you are on your back.

Falling asleep sitting on the lounge is also bad for your spine, as it doesn't allow for the discs to decompress at all and is bad for your leg circulation. Lying asleep on the average lounge isn't much better because the part you sit on is often sloped slightly backward so people do not slide forward onto the floor. This twists your spine, which can irritate your discs.

3.6   POSTURE AND WORK

Good posture helps breathing, digestion and circulation, as well as keeping your bones straight and strong. Good posture is kind of a continuous low-intensity strength exercise.

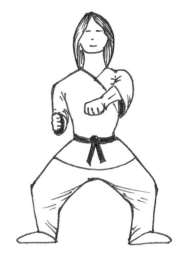

Posture is taken seriously in martial arts. The stances are the very first things taught because they give you better balance, power and movement. A chef friend of mine used his Kung Fu footwork to move around his kitchen when work got busy. He claimed it always helped him work faster and more efficiently. No air-kicks or shadow boxing, just nimble pivoting from one side of the kitchen to the other.

Most jobs do not contribute to good posture. You can mitigate at least some of the negative effects with the right exercises. Sit-down office and driving jobs, for instance, can have a shortening effect on your quads and hip flexors, so make a point of frequently stretching the muscles in the front of your thighs.

You can also use ergonomic seating. Saddle chairs are now very popular with dentists, who often have to contend with working at posturally difficult angles. Saddle chairs allow your legs to hang lower than normal chairs, forming a more comfortable hip/leg angle. As the name suggests, they are modeled on horse saddles.

Alas, the height of the average desk will not fit a saddle chair beneath. The opposite applies to sitting on a Swiss ball, which is usually too low for the average desk. Whatever form of seating you opt for, choose the one that will cause you the least problems. Sitting 40 hours a week, 48 weeks a year over your full working life can get hard on your back, so take regular stretching breaks.

Operating heavy power tools, tiling floors, digging holes, fixing overhead lights and pipes, cleaning and gardening can all be physically and posturally hard. Working predominantly with one hand can really create a right/left strength imbalance in your body.

To counter this state of affairs, you can help yourself by extra stretching for the muscles on the side of your body you use most and extra strengthening on the side you use least. Try to be as ambidextrous as safety and productivity allow you to be, and use lots of Self Massage.

4 STRETCHING

Stretching tends to be neglected more than cardio and strength training. When I was a regular gym user, I would see plenty of people do the weights and cardio and completely ignore the stretching area.

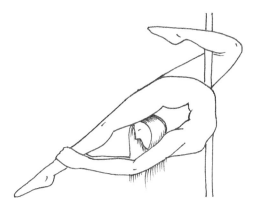

In recent years, we in Western countries are starting to warm up to the benefits of stretching, perhaps because of greater cultural contact with Asia, where the most recognizable stretching traditions come from.

When muscles are never stretched, they gradually shorten. When this happens, the joints that these muscles span can no longer fully open or close. We lose the joints' natural range of motion. The muscles and joints both suffer when stretching is not performed.

In the 1980's, I worked for a year in a nursing home. The elderly men and women were so stiff in their movements that it made a deep impression on me. Their legs, arms, hands, feet, necks and bodies moved like they were made of tin. I felt uncomfortable just watching them and I have done yoga ever since because the prospect of ever getting like that spooked me. I am going to do my best to spook you into it too.

If you are not naturally good at stretching, you will not help yourself by avoiding it. It may assist you if you take the attitude that it's like a necessary but foul-tasting medicine.

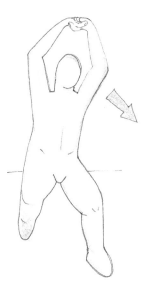

It is equally true of all types of exercise that those individuals who need it most are the least likely to do it. Even worse, progress with stretching is usually slow compared to the progress that can be made with strength training and cardio. Patience and persistence are required.

Well-stretched bodies move with greater ease, comfort and safety.

In yoga, stretching can become a type of meditation – it really does seem to work on the body and mind at the same time. Like tai chi and qigong (also known as chi gung), yoga can be performed for your whole life. If yoga is what you choose to get more flexible with, there is a lot to choose from.

More important than the actual style of yoga you learn is finding the right teacher. If the teacher has experienced similar physical challenges as you and is of a similar age, they are more likely to be on your wavelength. It can be hard for a younger teacher to imagine how much a body can tighten with chronic stretching neglect, dehydration and aging. Greater care is required with aging bodies.

Any yoga pose (asana) that causes pain should be avoided.

4.1   THE CONVENIENCE OF STRETCHING

Precious little space and absolutely no equipment is required to stretch – just two square meters of rug space to pad your ankles and knees. If you cannot easily get down to and back up off the floor, there are plenty of stretches you can do sitting or standing. A firm bed or level couch may be suitable too.

The stretching exercises that I present in this book have been picked because they are easy to do in a variety of settings, or because they involve several muscle groups at the same time, making them time-efficient.

Balance is paramount when stretching. It is very difficult to relax into a thorough stretch if you feel like you are about to tip over.
Sitting or lying on the floor is usually the best practice when stretching. If you can't get down to stretch and must stand, be sure that you are well supported, steady and well balanced.

At the time of writing this book, warm-up stretching before working out is widely regarded as being of no benefit. Post-exercise stretching, however, is desirable, especially when each stretch is held for a minimum of 20 seconds.

4.2   GETTING STRETCH-READY

Self Massage can help press out the kinks in your muscles to not only make stretching more comfortable but also to get results faster. Massage can also help free up scar tissue adhesions from old muscle trauma, making stretching much smoother and more enjoyable.

Repetitions are important in strength training but with stretching it is more beneficial to do one long stretch (20 seconds plus) rather than doing several shorter stretches. Cardio and strength exercise increase your heart rate, while stretching slows it down and calms the mind.

Any time of day is a good time to stretch. Cats, dogs and birds do it before and after napping. Their muscles are not unlike ours.

As with all exercise (strength and cardio), be attentive to your posture when stretching.

Part of the reason why so few of us are truly upright most of the time is because of the way we use our bodies in the workplace. If you are sitting down at a desk or if you drive all day, your body is continually bent forward. This has a shortening effect on the muscles at the front of your body, and is why we feel like we want to lean backward in our chairs so often.

Stretching doesn't just involve your larger muscles like your hamstrings. Your hands and fingers like to be stretched too. Anywhere you have muscle can do with some stretching.

4.3   PASSIVE STRETCHING

In passive stretching, you relax and let someone else stretch your muscles. This practice is commonplace in elite training because it is a more thorough and effective way to stretch. But unless your training partner is skilled and experienced with passive stretching, do **not** do it. This is not a task for novices. If your partner doesn't know when to stop, your muscles will tear.

Passive stretching is used often in bodywork. Good massage therapists, physiotherapists, osteopaths and chiropractors are all educated on how to do it. Passive stretching is used regularly on comatose and restricted mobility patients in order to prevent muscular contractures, a severe form of muscular shortening.

Like active stretching, passive stretching may work better after massage or Self Massage.

4.4   Stretching after injury

If you have had a moderate to severe muscle tear, it can be a while before you can attempt stretching that muscle again. Do it too soon or too fast and you will reinjure yourself.

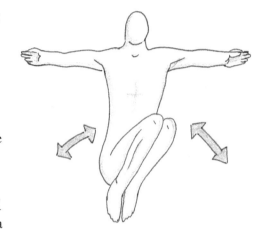

Overstretching is easy to do. I did it once during an adductor stretch when I was attempting straddle splits. It took me three months to get back to where I was before I injured myself.

If you have injured yourself, ease yourself gradually back into working the affected muscle. It is still OK to continue to exercise unrelated muscles – part of a workout is better than no workout at all.

Some Self Massage will help too. Work as close to the injury site as comfort will allow. If it feels touchy even with mild pressure, you are too close. In that case, move a little further away from the injury site and gently stroke away from it. As the pain and swelling goes away, you can progressively Self Massage with firmer pressure closer to the injury site.

When comfort allows, you can recommence stretching as you would when stretching for the first time. Continue to Self Massage the muscle, as this will help free any remaining internal adhesions left from the healing process.

4.5   Stretching and mirrors

It is OK to stretch in front of a mirror – in fact, it is the best way to compare your stretching posture to that of your teacher's. If you don't think it looks right, change your angle and analyze it. Even a slight change in the angle at which you are stretching can mean the difference between feeling awkward and feeling like you can relax into it and have gotten it just right. Don't just go through the motions of stretching – do them properly. Be persistent and be patient for results.

If you stretch regularly but cease improving, you may need to change your routine, do some Self Massage, or get treatment from a bodyworker.

5 CARDIOVASCULAR TRAINING

Cardiovascular training, or just *cardio*, is about getting into a low intensity rhythm of breathing and motion that raises your heart rate. Regular cardio can lower blood pressure, improve your stamina and ability to cope with sudden stress, reduce the chance of diabetes, improve circulation and create more oxygen-carrying red blood cells. It also shortens muscle recovery time, improves energy storage, increases muscle mass, reduces body fat and gives you real mental health benefits.

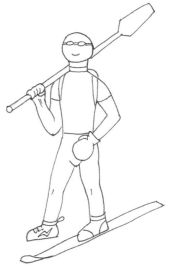

> *20 minutes of cardio, three times a week, has widely been recognized as the minimum requirement for a long while now. Even so, 5 or 10 minutes here and there is better than nothing at all.*

Most cardio involves leg-work like running, walking and cycling, but there is upper body cardio too: rowing, boxercise and swimming. Even if you are paraplegic, there are options.

Whatever cardio you do, be sure to always warm up. You can do this with Percussive Self Massage, walking or skipping. Then warm-down with stretching or more Self Massage.

At the age of 40, cartilage is starting to wear, so low impact cardio is best if you want to avoid joint pain. Recovery from big physical effort also takes longer post-40, so don't get discouraged if it takes a little longer for those after-exercise aches to fade than when you were 25.

It is best to mix cardio with stretching and strength exercises, as they help and complement one another. You may have a strong preference for one over the other, but they are all important.

Be realistic when buying gym membership or equipment. If you don't really like running or rowing, you probably won't use that treadmill or rower that you just paid hundreds for. If gym junkies annoy you, joining one makes no sense.

Cardio doesn't have to cost you anything at all if you are resourceful and earnest. If you like music, maybe dancing is best for you. If you like a laugh as you sweat it out, tape pictures of faces you don't like to your boxing pads. If your backyard pool is only 10 meters long, it doesn't matter that you need to do more turns, it is still good cardio. Work with whatever is available and motivates you.

If you choose your exercises wisely and do them properly, you will avoid injuries. I don't mean just the obvious mishaps like twisting an ankle but also the repetitive strain injuries from progressive accumulated muscle and joint micro trauma, such as from running on hard surfaces too often. Exercise smart by thinking carefully about what you are trying to achieve and how to get there before you start.

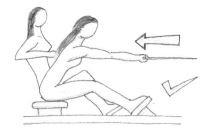

Whatever cardio you choose, be safe. Headphones get people run over – kind of a silly thing to do when you are trying to get fit. Showing off your sweaty body running on a hot day might attract people's attention for the wrong reasons (maybe they are only watching you because they are amused at why you are publicly dehydrating yourself). And always remember to drink more water when you exercise.

If you can only get to boot camp or spin class once a week, do some other cardio to supplement it. For example, wear your runners to work and walk hard to and from the bus stop. Wear a backpack instead of carrying a handbag or briefcase, as that will make walking much easier and more enjoyable. If you seek opportunities rather than excuses, you will find ways of fitting it in. Take the stairs at work, give junior a thrill with a brisk pram ride, or sit and do deep breathing exercises on the train. It all helps.

Even if you have a physical job, you should exercise anyway. Work activities typically involve a lopsided use of your body that distorts your posture, whereas exercise should be an even, posture-friendly physical activity.

If low physical energy is stopping you from exercising, discover the cause. Anemia, low thyroid function and insomnia are all treatable. Maybe your diet needs improvement. If you are asthmatic, learning Buteyko breathing may help your ability to do cardio.

5.1 BUTEYKO BREATHING

The first time I heard of Buteyko breathing was in a television documentary shot over several weeks in two medically supervised trials in hospitals in Bristol, UK and Brisbane, Australia. The participants were a group of male and female chronic asthma sufferers. The trial was conducted over several weeks and really did seem to help the people who stuck with it.

Those who participated reported easier breathing and better energy. I heard no comment from them about their emotional state, but to me they looked calmer. Many asthmatics get raised shoulder postures because of their rapid costal breathing. The shoulders of these people dropped to a lower more comfortable-looking level when they learned to breathe more slowly and deeply. They even looked more attractive.

Slower, deeper breathing has a natural calming effect because it doesn't stimulate the adrenals nearly as much as rapid shallow breathing. When we get emotionally excited, our breathing instantly becomes more rapid. Slowing the breath is a well-known method of stress management.

If you are under medical treatment for breathing problems, please discuss Buteyko breathing with your doctor before you try it.

Fortunately, Buteyko breathing is simple to learn. It is basically about taking deep breaths and holding them in for as long as you can as you slowly walk around. The objective is to increase your functional lung capacity. Even if you are not an asthmatic, you may find it beneficial to practice Buteyko breathing. It can be done for just a few minutes at a time in a variety of settings.

Buteyko breathing is not a cardio exercise in itself, but it may improve your ability to do cardio.

5.2 WALKING

An oldie but a goodie, walking is something nearly all of us can do to some extent. If you have no time for big walks, use your daypack and walk to the local grocery store instead of driving.

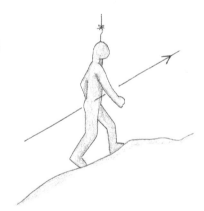

Walk in shoes that are comfortable to walk in. Change routes to keep it interesting, keep an upright posture and do it often. Swing your arms to walk faster.

Do it alone or with a friend, your dog or a group. Some good cardio before work or study can mentally sharpen your performance. Walking is an active meditation for many. In addition to being good cardio, it's good for your digestion, breathing, and leg and foot muscles.

Bushwalking is even better, as it gets that fine muscle control working in your feet, sidestepping rocks and roots. If you want to trek beyond pavement, take some ski stocks or at least a walking stick with you, as they will give you much better traction on steep loose climbs. They can also lessen impact on your knees during steep descents. **Go harder uphill and slower downhill.**

5.3 RUNNING

Running can be done almost anywhere. It is free and it is possible to lose weight quickly if you run **often**. The downsides are that joint pain can prevent you from running, or even be an effect of running.

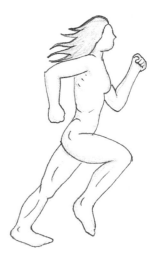

There are many choices to make for running: on the road, on grass, on the athletics track, on sand or running on the spot in shoulder-deep water. The road has highest joint impact and running in water the least.

What shoes to choose? Or go bare foot? Shoes protect your feet but twisting an ankle is rare when bare foot. Barefoot running enthusiasts believe that running with no shoes causes less shock through your skeleton because you are more likely to land on your mid-foot rather than your heel.

Day or night? It's harder to see in the dark but over-heating is less likely at nighttime.

What are you naturally best at? If you run as part of a group, is the pace to your liking? When running with others, there is peer pressure at work. Men in particular sometimes run too far as a group because of their competitive natures. If you are a natural sprinter, running short and sharp bursts in mini soccer, touch football or basketball may be a better fit for you than running miles along the road.

Orienteering can make running mid to longer distances more interesting with its navigation. There was even an attempt to popularize running between holes at golf some years back. There are many ways you can fit running into your life.

Avoid running downhill as it increases impact pressure on many joints in your body, particularly your leg joints. Running uphill has greater strengthening benefits and is easier on your joints.

This is too big a subject to deal with here in detail. Please consider the options to see what is the best fit for you, get unbiased advice about footwear, and start with shorter easy runs and gradually build up from there. Do not underestimate the importance of correct running technique. **Always run with even posture.**

If you feel a twinge running and cannot Self Massage or stretch the twinge out, you may need some assistance from a health professional. Sore knees that test negative for internal damage often respond well to Self Massage.

5.4 CLIMBING

Climbing is both cardio and a strengthening exercise for your arms, shoulders, back, hands and legs. It can offer a fast intense workout. Whether it is in the form of rock climbing, bouldering or mountaineering, climbing makes extensive use of all the muscles activated in chin-ups. The core muscles and leg muscles are used a lot too. A high power-to-weight ratio is a decided advantage – young children can be surprisingly good climbers.

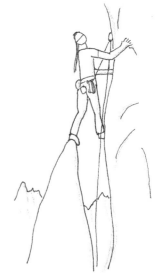

An important principle of exercise in general is to promote symmetrical muscle tone. Regular climbers have strongly favored sides, just like batters and pitchers. I never realized this until I massaged a few elite climbers; in each of them I found the muscles in their upper backs, though strong, were built up more on one side than the other. If you are a keen climber, it is good for your spine to even the strength up on the right and left sides of your back with other corrective exercises.

The muscles the hands grip with can be very strong in climbers, so regular Self Massage and stretching of the wrist flexors and hand muscles is very important in order to avoid RSI problems.

Climbing can be very hard on the fingertips, which can become numb and calloused, particularly on coarse rock. This can create problems if your occupation requires a high degree of sensitivity in the fingertips. Surgeons, osteopaths, chiropractors, massage therapists, jewelers and practitioners of fine arts can all be professionally disadvantaged by a loss of tactile acuity in their fingers.

5.5 SWIMMING AND AQUAROBICS

Swimming is mainly an upper body, low impact cardio exercise. It is much easier on your knees and back than running. All swimming strokes engage the muscles of your shoulders, upper back, forearms and to a lesser extent your legs. If you swim hard and fast, it becomes a strengthening exercise as well as cardio.

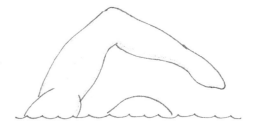

- **Freestyle (front crawl)** can be maintained for much longer than the other strokes so it is best for swimming longer distances. Freestyle is also good for stretching out a tight lower back. It will also firm your butt muscles more than the other strokes will. If you have difficulty with neck rotation, this stroke may aggravate it. If so, try Self Massaging your neck before swimming.

- **Breaststroke** uses the chest muscles most. If you want bigger and stronger chest muscles, it is your stroke of choice. If you have trouble rotating your head to look over your shoulder, breaststroke might be more comfortable than freestyle.
- **Backstroke** will stretch your spine out like freestyle does. Like breaststroke, it is easier on your neck than freestyle. If you are not a very confident swimmer and don't like your face underwater, it may be the best stroke for you. Please be careful about bumping your head on the end of the pool.
- **Butterfly** requires the most power, particularly in your upper back. The other strokes are more useful for cardio.

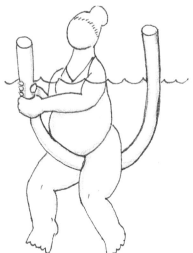

Aquarobics is also a good option for cardio exercise, particularly if you get hip, leg or foot pain from weight-bearing exercise. Many discover aquarobics through hydrotherapy while recovering from an operation.

More popular with women than men, aquarobics can be effective in sustaining leg strength and mobility when other exercise doesn't work. Aquarobics can be alternated with swimming.

5.6   BOXING AND MARTIAL ARTS

Boxing training (**boxercise**) is a great stress reliever and can improve your self-defense. Boxercise is good cardio and can help strengthen your upper body too. Alternate between left and right front foot stances for even muscle development. Do not punch heavy bags, as this can injure your hands and wrists.

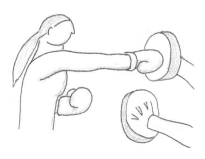

Martial arts **sparring** is also good cardio. When the patterns of movement are learned, the sparring becomes more like a synchronized dance than a brawl. If you learn judo, aikido or jiu jitsu, you will learn how to tumble safely when you fall over. This can help you avoid injury regardless of the cause of your fall. Find a martial arts teacher to whom you can relate.

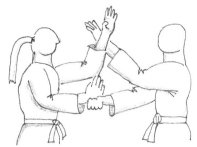

6 STRENGTH TRAINING

Several years ago, Balmain hospital in Sydney's Inner West hosted a course of supervised Progressive Resistance Training (with weights). Over a 6-week period, a group of men and women aged between 42 and 102 gathered to do this 3 times a week.

At the end of the 6 weeks, they all felt great and experienced performance and muscle mass increases between 15 and 90%. All the participants elected to continue their training at the end of the trial.

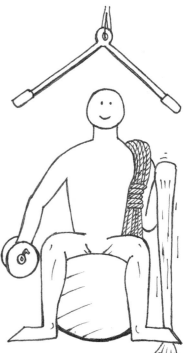

Strength training in your torso should always produce spine-straightening effects. Strength training done properly and regularly will improve your muscle, tendon and ligament strength. Muscle size, bone density, joint function, muscle recovery time, body shape and posture should all be improved by strength training.

In this book, a "rep" is a single lift, thus 10 reps is 10 lifts in a row. A "set" is the number of lifts (reps) in that row. Starting out lifting a lighter weight with a higher number of reps and then progressing to a heavier weight with fewer reps is called "tapering." This is a common and effective practice with strength training.

Because strength training is done by exerting your muscles against resistance such as weights or bands, it is also called resistance training. As you get stronger and gradually increase your weights, it is called PRT, for "progressive resistance training."

Posture is very important in strength training, as without good exercise posture (form), you will at best be ineffectual and at worst injured. If you do your strength training intelligently, it will in turn improve your posture.

Even though you may value your biceps or chest muscles above all others, even strength all over the body will give you not only good posture but attractive proportions as well.

Stretching and Self Massage is recommended after all strengthening exercises.

6.1   STRENGTH TRAINING & SPORT

One of the best contributions that strength training can offer the 40+ sportsperson is to promote symmetrical muscle strength in order to keep a straight spine. Tennis, baseball, shooting, and golf are all examples of sports that promote a lopsided muscularity in your back.

It is usually fairly obvious just by looking at a sportsperson's muscles what their strong side is. The greater the right/left strength disparity becomes, the more crooked it can eventually make the whole spine.

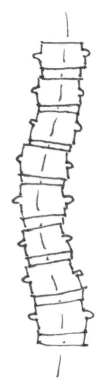

Look at the muscle anatomy drawings on the next page and in the Upper Body and Lower Body chapters. You will see that many muscles are fastened to different parts of the spinal column and are paired up right and left. Now imagine: what might happen to the position of the individual vertebrae (24 altogether) if the muscles on the right or left side of the spine are much stronger than the matching muscles on the other side?

When one level of the spine is deviated toward the stronger side, the body reacts by tensing muscles on the opposite side, at the levels above and below, in order to keep the body upright. This means that having uneven right/left strength at one level of your spine changes the strength balance at other levels of your spine too.

A good example of this is the relationship between your hips and shoulders. When viewed from above, your left shoulder moves forward as your right foot moves forward and vice versa. This way of moving produces torsion and therefore movement from the spine, as though it were a long steel spring.

Now imagine that your right shoulder is much stronger than your left, and how that might make your left hip muscles stronger than the right hip muscles. Watch what a right-handed baseball batter does with his left hip and thigh when he slams that ball – can you see the power in that action and how it might affect his spine in the long term?

Resistance training helps make your body more symmetrical by working it evenly. It can therefore help counter lopsidedness created by sport and work. Good form requires a straight spine.

6.2 AGONIST AND ANTAGONIST

Some bodybuilders have a tendency to work mainly on those muscles that they can see in the mirror, and neglect other muscles. This practice can give those individuals not only the muscles of a gorilla but the posture of one too. This is bad for your joints.

When you pitch a tent, it stands up best if the strings are evenly tensioned. So too it is with your postural muscles. While it can be a real confidence-builder getting impressive chest, shoulder and arm muscles – and there is nothing wrong with that – just remember the agonist/antagonist relationship of your muscles.

For example, when you are bending your arm at the elbow, the agonist is the biceps, and the antagonist is the triceps, which has the opposite action of straightening the elbow. It is good for your elbow to have a good strength balance between these two opposing muscles.

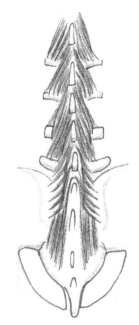

This same relationship exists between the front and back muscles of your thigh (quads and hamstrings), your lower leg (tibialis and calves), your upper body (upper chest and upper back muscles), and so on.

This principle applies to all your muscles. You will get much more pleasing results from strength training if you make a point of keeping things even.

6.3 FREE WEIGHTS VERSUS LIFTING MACHINES

Two common ways to get resistance training in a gym are with free weights and lifting machines. They both have important pros and cons.

Free weights give a more time-efficient workout because the helping or synergizing muscles – all those muscles that help the prime-moving muscle – are engaged. In a home gym situation, free weights are also cheaper and require less room.

Lifting machines are less time efficient to use and are bulkier and more expensive than free weights, but are safer. Synergizing muscles such as the upper trapezius and wrist flexors and extensors can easily get overused when free weights are used a lot. This can give you wrist, elbow and neck pain. Lifting machines are less likely to do this.

A lot of more serious looking exercisers with lifting belts and big muscles tend to use the gym free weights rooms, but don't let that fool you. You can get just as strong working with the machines. It just might take a little longer.

Free weights feel like they weigh the same anywhere, while lifting machines can feel different from machine to machine because of differences between brands. Take this into account if you work out in different gyms. It is not a good idea getting too fixated on the numbers on the iron – how it feels to you is more important.

6.4   SPOTTING

Spotting is when you work with a partner during weight training. The idea is that they stand there ready to help you if you bite off more than you can chew and suddenly find yourself losing control of a lift. Losing control is most dangerous when you are bench-pressing a heavy weight, and it can be fatal if your strength gives out with the bar across your throat.

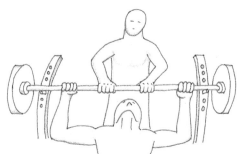

I and another person literally walked into an otherwise empty weights room one day to find someone in the process of losing control of a throat-bound bench press. Needless to say, this otherwise strong-looking man was grateful to us for showing up when we did. Quite fittingly, we were there for a fitness leader weight training class.

If you want to be adventurous with free weights and test your limits, do it with a spotter, never alone. Remember also that you must wait about two minutes between sets before you have full power again for the next lift.

6.5   FAST-TWITCH AND SLOW-TWITCH MUSCLE FIBER

Fast-twitch and slow-twitch muscle fiber is also called white and red muscle fiber. In a chicken, for example, there is more red muscle fiber in the legs because red slow-twitch muscle is more suited to low-speed walking. The wings and breast muscles in chickens are white fast-twitch fiber, which is essential for the more rapid muscle action that enables flight.

Not all of us are made with the same red/white muscle fiber balance. People who are good sprinters tend to have more white muscle fiber and these people get bigger muscles faster than those who have more red muscle fiber. Red muscle fiber is more suited to endurance sports. Think of how sprinters and marathon runners look so different to one another.

If you come from a long line of red-fiber slow-twitch ancestors, you will find it more difficult to bulk up. I have known red-fiber dominant men who cannot bulk up no matter how hard they try. I have known white-fiber dominant women who get bigger muscles with relatively little effort. It all comes down to our genes.

The good news is that even if you cannot get big muscles, you can still achieve good muscular definition by achieving a low fat to body mass index when you work out.

Please remember that muscle weighs more than fat, so you may lose inches rather than weight as the lighter fat cells shrink and the denser muscle cells grow.

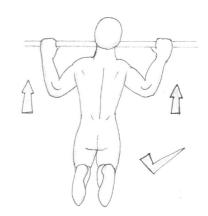

Weights and resistance training are great if you stick to the rules of good lifting. But never overlook the simple stuff like push-ups, chin-ups and squats, and low-tech equipment like Thera-Bands.

6.6 CHEATING

Cheating – as the name suggests – is not good. Cheating is when you distort your posture (use poor form) and/or shorten your lifting action in order to move a heavier weight or achieve increased repetitions, instead of using the target muscle strength alone. Cheating can mean bending your spine into potentially injurious postures under load or shortcutting full extension and contraction of the target muscle.

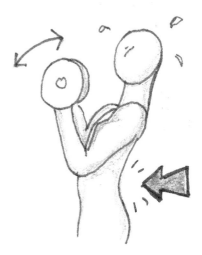

Cheating can give you back injuries and tendonitis, which are painful, restrictive and slow to heal.

We all have limitations, so be honest with yourself. Getting obsessed with personal bests can really mess you up and be very counterproductive. Pay attention to how you are feeling while you are exercising rather than obsessing about time and measurements.

6.7 RESISTANCE TRAINING AND MIRRORS

The mirrors in gyms are not there just for vanity. If possible, directly face a full-length mirror while you are doing weights, as it is the best way of checking your form. If you don't look even, you may need to drop the weight on the bar a little. Always lift evenly.

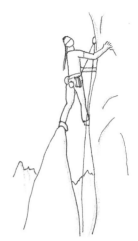

If you favor rock climbing as your chief resistance exercise, mirrors are not terribly useful. Any exercise that you cannot see yourself do is best observed and critiqued by someone with expertise. Be open to criticism, as it is the best way to achieve good technique.

6.8 STRENGTH TRAINING OUTSIDE THE GYM

Weights can be very rewarding to work with if you are thinking about what you are doing and why. You don't have to use weights for resistance training, though, as there are convenient alternatives.

Thera-Bands, for example, are used a lot in Pilates and are very light, inexpensive and portable. I always carry a pair around in my daypack. They are color-coded according to their differing strengths. Despite being very useful, they tend to be underutilized by men.

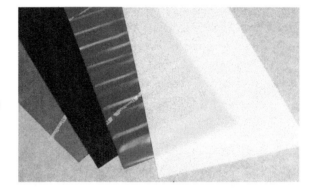

If you are strong, you can use two Thera-Bands at once. **Please do not improvise with non-purpose-made elastic products such as luggage straps, as they can cause serious injury.**

In many parks you will now find exercise stations. Most of the strengthening exercises in this book don't need equipment or a lot of space to perform. Keeping exercise simple and portable makes it more effective.

If you work out regularly but cease to improve, you need to change your workout routine.

If you do bulk up more than you feel comfortable with, stick more with the cardio and stretching. Sometimes women worry about getting big muscles if they use weights. But unless you have an unusually high level of male hormones in your body or have a high proportion of fast-twitch muscle fiber (or use growth promoters), this is unlikely to happen.

7 FUNCTIONAL FITNESS

For a long time, physical fitness was widely defined as having good measures of flexibility, strength and cardio stamina. Now there is a fourth category: functional fitness, also called neuromotor fitness. The importance of functional fitness increases as we age.

Think about what you do when you need to quickly clean up a room, reaching to dust, bending to sweep, darting from one side of the room to the other, side-stepping furniture as you go. You engage hundreds of muscles to do these things, and as long as you can do them for yourself you don't need anyone else to do them for you. **Neuromotor exercise** combines stretching, strengthening and cardio to engage muscles in whole body movements.[1]

Posture, **agility**, **balance** and **proprioception** (position awareness), are neuromotor catchwords. When your posture is good, your body looks and feels better. When you have good agility you move better. If you are well balanced you are better able to avoid accidents and injuries. Proprioception is your awareness of your own movement – it has a lot to do with thinking about **how** you are moving.

Functional fitness has its origins in physical and occupational therapy. Helping patients to recover from surgery, sickness and trauma to return to their homes and jobs has been their focus for decades.

Functional fitness is not the same for everybody. For example, a hospital patient returning to a home with many steps will need more stair climbing practice than a patient returning to a step-free environment. Functional fitness physically adapts us to the demands of our surroundings. It is increasingly topical because populations in many countries are aging, and there is a real fear that in the near future there will not be enough young to look after the old. This means that the elderly will have to get better at looking after themselves.

The positive of this situation is that becoming a fitter and more active elderly person, whatever the reason, is a good thing. Elderly people suffer terribly when they lose their independence and mobility. Functional fitness is an important health and lifestyle intervention that you can do to help yourself remain independent.

---

[1] Please note that housework itself is no substitute for neuromotor exercises, as the exercises have much more wide-ranging benefits than making your chores easier.

7.1 NEUROMOTOR EXERCISE

In neuromotor exercise, you consciously match exercises to tasks. For example, squatting exercises help us to get onto and off chairs safely and easily. Many elderly people have accidents trying to sit or stand, or break bones trying to get on and off toilets. You should be physically able to stop and hold your position without falling backward or forward whenever you are getting onto or off a chair. If you don't have the necessary strength or control in your legs to do this, you cannot stop yourself from lowering your full bodyweight onto something dangerous, like a wine glass you didn't see (for instance).

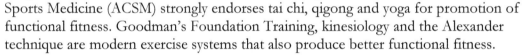

There are exercise systems, both ancient and modern, that are good for functional fitness. The American College of Sports Medicine (ACSM) strongly endorses tai chi, qigong and yoga for promotion of functional fitness. Goodman's Foundation Training, kinesiology and the Alexander technique are modern exercise systems that also produce better functional fitness.

The regular practice of such exercise systems will help you avoid events like falling and breaking your hip, a common life-shortening occurrence for many elderly people. Prevention is way better than cure – it is much better to get into good exercise habits in your 40's than to panic about your fitness in your 70's or 80's.

If you are getting weak and losing your balance, it is a trap to play it safe by staying sitting in a nice comfortable chair all day. The more people do this, the weaker and more accident-prone they become. Incontinence can also be a result of weakening leg and hip muscles.

Simple things like being able to get down on the floor and play with your kids and grandkids are helped by doing neuromotor exercise. You can avoid embarrassment by remaining functionally fit. It is much more enjoyable being able to help someone else up off the ground than needing it yourself.

Core muscle strength is central to functional fitness. This illustration of Goodman's bending down exercise is a good example of balance combining with strength with a straight spine to enable everyday activities like pulling weeds or mopping up a spilt drink. Lowering your body this way takes the strain out of bending your back and spares your knees the discomfort of kneeling down and squatting.

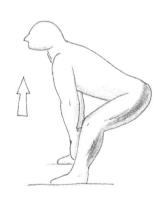

Look at the Goodman's exercises later in this chapter. Like tai chi, the stances are always wide. This is not only good for balance, but it is much easier to keep a straight spine with widely spaced feet. You can feel your legs getting stronger with Goodman's exercises. This increasing leg strength spares your back from bending so much, and means better functional fitness because aging knees cannot squat and kneel like they once did.

Yoga can improve your functional fitness too, particularly with the upright asanas (poses). There are many asanas in ashtanga yoga and bikram yoga (hot yoga) that strengthen postural muscles and improve balance. Not all asanas are easy to do, however, and some – like headstands and the cobra pose – I don't recommend at all to people over 40.

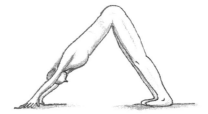

Asanas like the one at right, the "downward dog," can help strengthen your core as you stretch your hamstrings and calves. Yoga teachers will often get you to do breathing exercises as you go through the moves. Slowing the breath as you stretch not only makes stretching easier, but also calms the mind.

You need very little room or equipment to do yoga, just a mat to sit or lie down on. It is very economical, portable and simple.

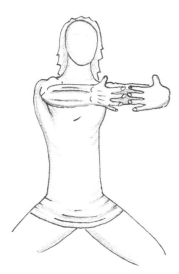

Qigong is another functional exercise system that is portable and easy on space. Qigong is tai chi's lesser-known cousin. It is practiced in slow motion like tai chi but unlike tai chi, it doesn't look like a martial art. Qigong looks more like mime than slow combat practice. Breathing exercises and color visualization tend to be utilized more in qigong than in tai chi.

Qigong strengthens postural muscles; it is focused precision movement like tai chi. To slowly execute the curved movements can be very exacting on your muscles, but the movements become more fluid as the muscles strengthen.

Perhaps there is some mind over matter involved but as you get better at doing qigong (and tai chi too), it feels as though you are pushing against an unseen force.

Teachers of tai chi and qigong will often tell their students to feel for this unseen gentle resistance. This training method may provide researchers important clues about how tai chi and qigong works.

Although qigong looks a lot less like a martial art than tai chi, it seems to attract the attention of martial artists more. While it is beyond the scope of this book to speculate about the deeper powers that qigong is said to tap into, I can vouch for my personal experience of it. Qigong really feels like it lifts my energy each time I do it.

The portability of these exercise systems is ideal for today's smaller urban abodes. Tai chi, yoga and qigong are totally relevant to the most modern lifestyle.

It is much easier to learn tai chi, yoga and qigong from a teacher than from any book. Videos are the next best thing, particularly for tai chi and qigong. Don Fiore has some short tai chi and qigong videos online at www.youtube.com, which are quite good at showing the basics to beginners. For yoga, most of the free online instruction I have found is too advanced for beginners, so it is best to find a good teacher, at least to start with.

Starting on page 45, I list five neuromotor exercises recommended by Kinesiology Professor Dr. Barbara Bushman. You may look at these and think, "They are for oldies, not me." It is easy to laugh at these simple exercises right up until the day you can no longer do them. So I invite you to just try them for yourself to see how well you can do them. They are simple but important, because as long as you can still do them, you are less likely to fall over and seriously injure yourself.

Starting on page 47, I list six exercises from Dr. Eric Goodman's Foundation Training. Goodman's Foundation Training helps you straighten your back by strengthening your core muscles. If you look at these exercises and think, "How is that going to help me?", you are not alone. I thought so too at first, but when I started to see the results, it won me over. I have directed several of my massage and acupuncture clients to this training and they found it just as useful as I did.

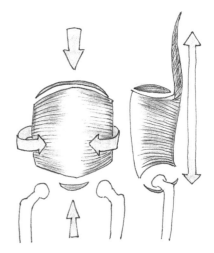

The exercises listed here will only take you a few minutes. Goodman's full exercise program is bigger than this but these few exercises will help you to better core strength. Even doing these few correctly and often may surprise you with how much they reduce back pain and improve your posture. You can find good instructive videos on Dr. Goodman's website, www.foundationtraining.com.

The term "neuromotor" does have a bit of a robotic ring to it, but it is really about doing quite normal things in the most balanced, agile, proprioceptive and posturally correct way possible.

Try the exercises in this chapter even if you think they look too easy to even bother trying. The first sign that you need to do such exercises is finding them challenging when you attempt them.

7.2 FIVE NEUROMOTOR EXERCISES

M1 Tube pick up

This simple exercise helps you to maintain and improve the fine motor function of your feet while improving your balance. Stand near something solid enough to steady yourself on, and pick up a cardboard tube with your toes. Then drop it and pick it up again from wherever it lands. Repeat several times, and then do the other foot.

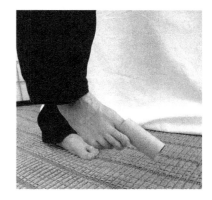

M2 Pretend sits

This exercise is about thigh strength, balance and muscular control. As legs weaken, people start flopping themselves down on chairs, surrendering control of the most powerful muscles in the body. This is a safety issue: if you accidentally sit on something dangerous like a wine glass, you can stand up again straight away if your descent is controlled. But if your butt is in free fall, those last few inches can cause serious injury.

As you can see from the photograph, the spine is kept straight. Ease yourself from standing down to hovering an inch or two above the seat. Hold this position for a few seconds and then stand again. Repeat several times. **This exercise is as functional as it gets and should be practiced by everybody over 40**.

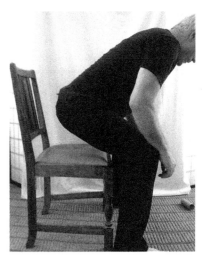

M3 Sock stand

Stand barefoot and put your socks on and take them off again a few times each side. This is a good test for the fine muscle balance control in the soles of your feet. When we walk on flat level surfaces all the time, the small but potentially strong muscles in your soles get lazy. Poor balance lessens your agility. Repeating this task improves your balance.

If you wear socks or stockings most days, this is an easy exercise to add to your normal routine.

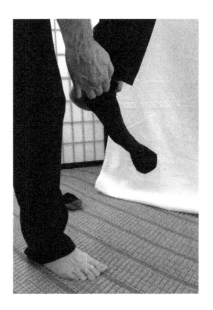

M4   Ball toss

Ball toss can be done sitting or standing. Toss a ball from one hand to the other, alternately catching and tossing each side. As it gets easier, increase the toss height and move your hands further apart. If that's easy, toss standing up or even balanced on one leg at a time.

This exercise assists neural crossover between the two sides of your brain. It assists coordination and encourages ambidextrousness. This in turn helps to promote even muscle development between the right and left sides of your body.

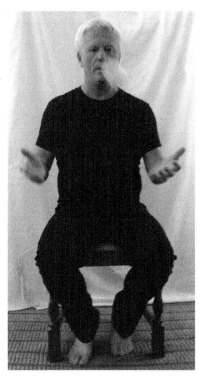

M5   Bushwalking

Bushwalking can improve your functional fitness. Stepping over tree roots, fallen branches, between and on top of rocks helps your cardiovascular function, balance and agility. All as you take in the beauty, air, sounds and fragrances of nature. Bushwalking is a good cardio and neuromotor exercise.

The functional application of bushwalking is to assist your ability to safely react to obstacles in your path and to give you better spatial awareness. Familiar surroundings make us complacent and inattentive – most accidents occur in the home.

If you feel vulnerable being out alone in a secluded place, join a bushwalking group. Local newspapers, magazines and community notice boards advertise bushwalking groups.

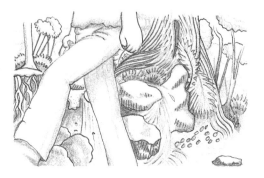

7.3   SIX GOODMAN'S EXERCISES

M6   Starting position

With your feet a shoulder's width apart, back straight and knees very slightly bent, place your hands on your waist. Keep your thumbs touching the bottom of your rib cage and your pinkies touching the top of your pelvis to ensure your back remains straight.

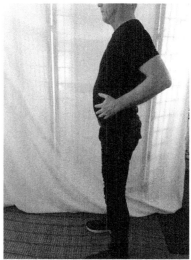

The purpose of this exercise is to learn to lean forward and backward from your hips. Take your weight through your heels while keeping a straight back. Suck your belly in.

As you lean forward, extend your butt backward and your chest forward. Your knees should be slightly behind your ankles when viewed side-on.

If your thumbs and pinkies remain in their starting position, it ensures that your back remains straight and your weight is going through your heels. All forward and backward movement comes from your rotating hip joints. Your hamstrings, butt and calves should feel like they are doing all the work as you tip backward and forward.

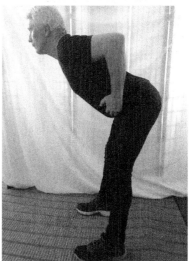

Repeat several times.

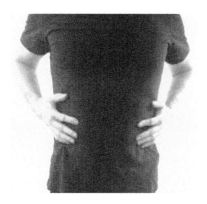

M7   Rolling shoulder stretch

Stand up straight with your feet a shoulder's width apart and with a slight bend in your knees. Tuck your chin in and suck your belly in. Roll your shoulders backward a few times. This helps straighten and relax your upper body and readies you for core exercise.

Don't roll your shoulders forward: this will make you slouch forward.

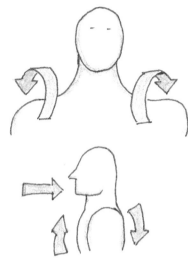

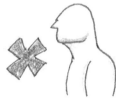

M8   Founder posture

Stand with your feet a shoulder's width apart. Take your weight through your heels as you lean forward from your hips. Push your butt backward to maintain your head's position directly above your heels. With your chin in, belly sucked in, pelvic floor tensed and back straight, start with your arms by your side as shown. Turn your palms out so that your thumbs face upward.

Inhale deeply as you raise your arms forward and above your head. As you raise your arms, move your butt further backward to maintain your balance. When viewed side-on, your knees should be slightly bent and behind your ankles. Exhale as you drop your arms to return to the starting position. Do as many reps as you can at a controlled pace until you tire.

When you get this exercise right, you will feel the muscles in your butt and at the back of your legs do all the work. If you feel any strain at all in your back, stop and check to find out what you are doing wrong.

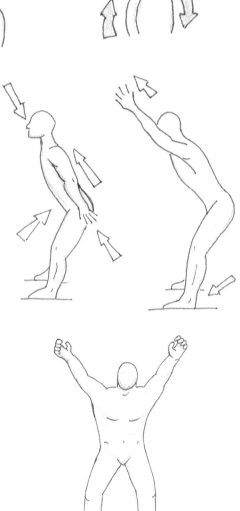

M9 Bending down

Start in the Founder posture: belly tensed, weight through heels, chin tucked in, chest out, pelvic floor tensed, butt out, back straight. Raise your arms, then lower your fingertips to the floor and exhale as you do so. If your knees don't bend well, this is a good way to weed your garden or pick up coins. Run your hands up your legs as you stand back up. Repeat until you tire.

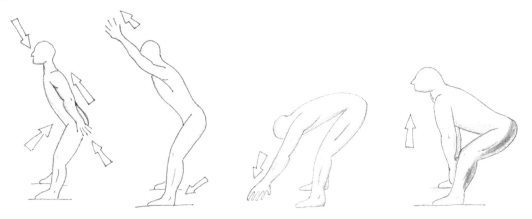

As before, inhale as you raise your arms and exhale as you lower them. This exercise is a good example of how Goodman's exercises teach us to lower and raise the body from the hips instead of bending the back.

M10 The woodpecker

Place one foot forward and the other back. Keep your belly sucked in, chin in, back straight, forward foot slightly forward of the knee, rear heel off the floor, and pelvic floor flexed (as though were stopping yourself from peeing). Inhale as you raise your arms forward and upward. Your upper body leans forward slightly so your head is above the forward knee. Hold this position for a few seconds and exhale as you lower your arms. Do both sides and repeat until tired.

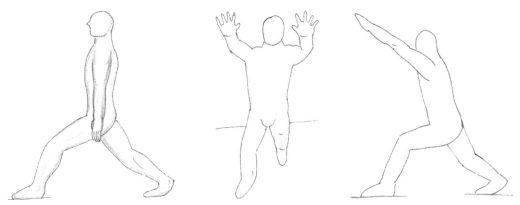

M11 Stretching up

Place one foot forward and the other back. Raise your hands above your head and interlock your fingers with your palms facing up. Keep your back straight, pelvic floor tensed, belly sucked in, rear heel raised, front foot slightly forward of the knee, and chin tucked in. Then lean backward and to the side away from the rear foot (for example, if your right foot is back, lean backward and to the left).

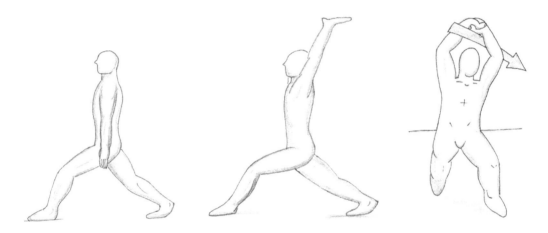

Inhale as you stretch back and sideways. You should feel your upper thigh stretch in this position. Hold this position until tired, and then do the other side. Exhale as you drop your arms.

Goodman's Foundation Training videos on www.youtube.com are quite instructive. The postural exercises shown here are just a few of his full range of exercises. All six Goodman's exercises shown are core strengthening and are a good alternative to planking if you have difficulty getting down onto the floor.

8 ACHES & PAINS

Pain is a natural distress signal that warns the brain that the body it is in danger of being damaged. Our ability to sense pain is there for our own protection.

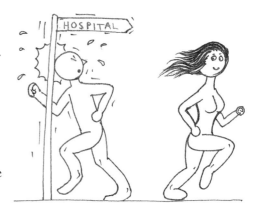

There are important qualitative differences in types of pain, such as intensity, sharp or dull, and so on. A low level of dull pain, for instance, is a normal feeling when exercising hard or getting a firm massage. Sharp pain, on the other hand, is not a normal exercise or massage sensation and should be avoided; it is a warning of impending damage.

Pain can be masked by the presence of pain-killing drugs as well as body hormones. Endorphins and encephalins are naturally produced by the body when you are working or playing hard.

If you are injured while under the influence of pain-killing drugs or hormones, you will usually not feel the full pain until the hormones or drugs have worn off a few hours later. This is why it is important that, if you feel like something painlessly gives way and suddenly weakens during a strenuous physical activity, you stop immediately. Continuing at even a reduced intensity will probably worsen the damage in the joint or muscle.

Working through the "pain barrier" is a job for highly trained athletes who know their limitations, not for people trying to get fit again. Any sharp pain or strong dull pain is a definite warning to back off from what you are doing.

8.1 SPRAINS AND STRAINS

A *sprain* is a ligament injury. Ligaments are the fibrous tissue sheets that join bones to one another at the joints. A severe sprain causes joint instability and occurs when the joint is hyperextended (stretched past its normal range of motion).

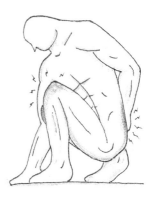

Twisting your ankle playing soccer is a good example of how a sprain can occur.

A *strain* is a muscle or tendon injury that occurs as the result of over-exertion or the hyperextension of a muscle. A severe strain can completely detach a muscle from the bone, either at the tendon where the muscle is fastened to the bone or through the middle of the muscle. Both can have a deforming effect on the shape of the muscle.

Tearing your Achilles tendon shooting a basket is a good example of how strains can occur.

It is possible to do both at the same time with severe trauma, but fortunately they both require the same first aid: ice. They are both painful and require medical examination.

Generally speaking, muscles tend to heal quickly because they are highly vascular (contain a lot of blood vessels), whereas tendon, ligament and cartilage tend to be much slower to heal because they contain relatively few blood vessels. That is why they are white (as opposed to red muscle).

Even bone heals faster than tendon, ligament and cartilage because the marrow in its center is highly vascular and bone has little blood vessel tunnels through the hard walls.

8.2   HOT VERSUS COLD

The golden rule is to ice a fresh injury and to heat longer-term aches and pains.

It is most important to know when to use ice (cryotherapy) as opposed to heat (thermotherapy) for soft tissue pain. If you use ice on a muscle in an area of chronic (long term) pain it can make the symptoms worse. Likewise, using a hot pack on a fresh swollen injury is counter-productive too.

When first injured, apply a cold pack to the injured area. Ensure you wrap the cold pack in a small towel – do not apply the pack directly to your skin. After 10 to 20 minutes, remove the cold pack and allow the injured area to rest for 10 to 20 minutes. Then repeat. Continue icing like this for 4 to 6 hours, then ice 10 minutes per hour after that.

If the swelling has not subsided after three days, see your doctor. If coldness or inactivity makes your back or joints ache, warmth is best applied. Like cold packs, hot packs should be wrapped in a small towel and not put directly on your skin.

If you are in doubt about the appropriate first aid because of conflicting signs, seek the advice of a health professional.

8.3   MISLEADING PAIN SENSATIONS

Sometimes an injury can be hard to shake off because it keeps recurring. You may need to modify what you are doing or just resign yourself to requiring some form of regular therapy so you can keep exercising or playing. Self Massage can assist you with such problems.

Referred pain is a common obstacle to healing, because the sensations can give you misleading and confusing symptoms. For example, if you have a sore wrist or elbow that defies your best efforts at self-help, the problem could in fact be in your neck – which can be confusing if your neck doesn't feel sore. Pressure on the arm's nerve roots up in the neck can do this.

A lower back problem may produce leg pain without any back pain, and even though there is nothing at all wrong with your leg. Trusting your sense of touch alone will not always lead you to the right conclusions about what is going on inside your body:

> *When I was at university we were paired up and given skin fold calipers to do an experiment one night. We were not measuring each other's rolls of fat as the calipers are designed for, but to see how reliable the sense of touch is. We all took turns guessing whether the settings of the calipers were changed, relying on our sense of touch alone.*

> *When the calipers were gently pressed against the fingertips or lips, it was possible to detect a change in caliper width as little as 2 or 3 millimeters, but when applied to the back or thigh it was impossible to notice a change in the distance between the caliper jaws up to 90 millimeters. It was an excellent demonstration of sensory acuity – where there are many nerve endings, our sense of touch and pain is accurate. There are way more nerve endings in the fingertips than on the back and thighs.*

Stiff muscles adjacent to our joints can make the joints ache. The next time your knee, elbow or shoulder starts aching for no apparent reason, Self Massage the muscles all around the sore joint. Be sure to probe around and massage from all angles.

The tensions that stiff muscles can apply to a joint will often not feel like muscular pain at all, but rather a deeper, more intense and restrictive joint sensation. Our bodily sensations can be easy to misinterpret at times. Self Massage and exercise helps your mind to better familiarize itself with your body.

8.4 AUTOIMMUNE DISEASE

There are about 80 different autoimmune diseases. Not all of them produce muscle and joint problems, but the ones that do can be excruciatingly painful. Fibromyalgia, rheumatoid arthritis and polymyalgia rheumatica (PMR) are but three examples of these nasty unpredictable conditions.

Autoimmune diseases see the body's natural defenses, like the white blood cells, attack healthy tissue, mistaking it for harmful germs. Autoimmune diseases have an unknown cause, can strike without warning and can be very difficult to bring under control.

Autoimmune diseases can make most exercise and even your work impossible because of the pain.

The above conditions are mentioned here because they are much more prevalent from 40 onward. Most forms of cardio and resistance training will not be possible, but some of the stretches and Self Massage techniques in this book may be of value to you.

I have known people who have had little respite from these conditions over a number of years. My PMR was terrible for 12 months. After a great deal of osteopathy, massage, acupuncture, glucosamine, fish oil and recommended doses of paracetamol and a course of corticosteroids, 4 years later I feel completely recovered.

I am glad I tried so hard to get on top of it – if you or someone close to you has such a condition, don't give up. If you keep trying new things, you will learn how to help yourself. It is important to accept the fact that our bodies do not last forever and to take the view that health is a process, not a final destination.

8.5   BACK PAIN

A health study published several years ago showed that 70% of people who claimed they have never had lower back pain previously actually had disc prolapse. Disc prolapse is a bulging of the soft rubbery gel-filled discs between your vertebrae (backbones).

The discs act as shock absorbers and flexible joins in your back. When they wear down, dehydrate or become injured, your spine can get stiff, sore, and less resistant to shock.

Through heavy lifting, weight gain or doing something sudden and lopsided – like hitting a golf ball hard – your bulging disc that doesn't hurt can easily become one that does.

Disc prolapse ("slipped disc") and degeneration can cause severe back pain and sciatica (pain, numbness and/or tingling into your legs and/or groin). It can take you completely by surprise the first time it happens to you. It usually occurs for the first time while we are still young. It heals, but may leave a lasting weakness that can be re-injured later in life.

Fortunately, with professional treatment, back pain is usually treatable. **You must always lift with a straight spine because you do not know what hidden weaknesses may be inside.** You may get away with poor lifting technique for a while, but eventually you will suffer for it.

Posture is very important when you are doing resistance training. It is your best insurance against injuring yourself while you are doing it. **Form** is the word used to describe correct exercise posture.

8.6   SPORTS TRAUMA

There are some types of injury that are more commonly sustained on the sports field and in the gym. This does not mean, however, that sports injuries are entirely different to muscle and joint injuries sustained at work or in your home.

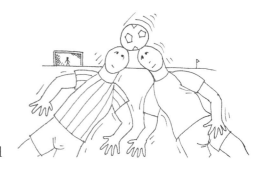

Sprains and strains to your ankle or knee are very common in sport, although you can just as easily stumble on a flight of stairs and sustain an identical injury.

A heavy lifting injury of your back, on the other hand, is more likely sustained at work or at home. You can also hurt your back weightlifting in the gym.

Be sensible and realistic about recovering from an injury. If you want best results, follow the advice of your therapist. Don't blame a slower-than-desired recovery on them if you do not follow his or her advice.

All other things being equal, the younger you are, the faster you recover. For best results, you should continue treatment until normal function returns – not just until the pain goes away. It will usually take longer to regain normal function, but the risk of re-injury is lower if the course of treatment is complete.

As the injured muscle heals, you can gently stroke away from the injury site at the edges of the swelling to try to speed things up a little. If you have injured one calf muscle, you should Self Massage the other calf too, because it will be working much harder than it usually does.

Ease the injured muscle back into exercise tentatively and after the bruising has subsided. Applying massage directly to the trauma site – when it is comfortable to do so – can help free any internal adhesions left from the healing process.

Just as you can see that new skin isn't exactly the same as it was before a cut or a graze, freshly healed muscle is not exactly the same as it was pre-injury either. This is called scar tissue and it usually responds well to stretching and massage, when judiciously applied. The edges of scar tissue can become weak points. Massage and stretching help prevent injury re-aggravation.

8.7   WHY DO I FEEL SORE?

If you are not used to strenuous exercise, it can steeply elevate lactic acid levels in your bloodstream and cause cramping, nausea and weakness. When you are still sore days later, it is more likely to be due to mild rhabdomyolosis (*rhabdo*) from traumatized muscle cells.

Mild rhabdo can also result from a very firm massage that leaves you feeling sore days later, as a result of rupture of muscle cells. Stiff and weak muscles are more likely to suffer mild rhabdo because individual muscle fibers rupture more easily, but in a less intense and dramatic way than a bigger muscle tear.

This type of mild rhabdo passes after a few days. You can avoid it by applying Self Massage and exercise *gradually*. As your body gets used to both, there is less incidence of traumatized muscle cells from either.

Overheating can cause rhabdo too. In extreme cases, "muscle meltdown" can permanently damage muscles and kidneys and even kill you. Please do not push yourself strenuously when exercising in hot conditions.

If you cramp easily, you may need a nutritional assessment to see if you are getting all the water, vitamins and minerals you need, as deficiencies can cause pain and weakness. Stress and lack of sleep can make you feel sore too, through raised cortisol hormone levels in your bloodstream.

Don't expect your body to perform as well as it did 20 years ago, and give it longer to recover from exertion.

9   SAFETY FIRST

Not everything in this book is for everyone. **If any of the activity described in this book causes pain, dizziness, nausea or shortness of breath, stop and check if you are doing it correctly.** If you are but are still struggling, move on to something else and see a physical therapist or doctor if it happens again the next time you try.

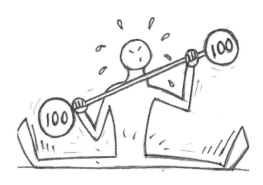

9.1   GENERAL SAFETY

- If you are being medically treated for any condition, let your doctor know you are trying to get fit.

- Do not physically exert yourself or Self Massage while under the influence of drugs or alcohol.

- Sharp or strong pain is a warning to back off. Pushing through the pain barrier can mask an injury through the body's natural painkillers being activated, and you may cause yourself further damage without realizing it till later.

- If you have sustained an injury that is still swollen and painful, give the muscle and skin a chance to heal before exercising or Self Massaging it again.

- It is important that you feel well balanced while performing any exercise or Self Massage technique.

- **Focus on what you are doing.** Fiddling with your iPod while you are running, for example, is an unsafe practice.

- Ensure that you always exercise in a suitable area that is free of clutter. A towel left lying on the floor can trip you over, for example, and slippery polished floors might make feet in socks skid.

- Pets and young children love pouncing on adults lying or sitting on the floor, so do your floor exercises and Self Massage when the kids are in bed and the dog is outside.

- Stretch SLOWLY, with no sudden jerks or bouncing. If you cannot relax into a stretch, you may be doing it incorrectly or trying too hard. It may also be that the stretch is too difficult for you at this point in time.

- Form is **everything**. The correct posture for each and every exercise and Self Massage technique is essential for safety and efficacy.

9.2 EXERCISE SAFETY

- Warm up before doing anything vigorous, particularly when cold.

- Hamstrings and calves can tear easily if you take off for a sprint and they are not used to it. Torn muscles can set you back weeks or even months. Stretching and massage can reduce the incidence of leg injury and help you to run better. Get at least one thorough massage before you intend on re-engaging in training after a layoff.

- An exercise that you found quite achievable yesterday may not feel as easy today. If in doubt, don't push it. Be conscious of your body feeling a little different from day to day.

- If you are even a little bit unsure about how a piece of exercise equipment works, ask someone who knows. Men like asking these questions as much as they enjoy asking pedestrians which street they are on. And certainly don't go giving pointers to anyone else who you think knows even less than you do.

- Be cautious about lifting weights over your head. These exercises can be tough on the shoulders and neck and have few benefits outside of contact sport and weightlifting competition.

- Unlawful exercise supplements are illegal for good reasons – don't use them.

- Just because someone looks fit does not mean they can make you look just like them, even if they are a qualified trainer. If you have little fast-twitch muscle fiber, it can be near impossible to build big muscles. If you come from a long line of ectomorphs (naturally skinny people), you may never bulk up, but achieving impressive muscle definition may still be perfectly attainable.

- Don't do something just because someone who looks strong is doing it. Strong-looking people make exercise mistakes too. It is sensible to research everything before you start.

- Muscle melt-down (rhabdomyolosis) is real – do not push yourself in hot conditions. The more you sweat, the more water you must drink to prevent dehydration and potential organ damage.

PART II

Self Massage and exercises for all areas of your body.

10 Neck & Jaw

Your neck is the most vulnerable section of your spinal column and needs to be treated with great care. Its muscular structure is complex, allowing great subtlety of movement that enables us to use our eyes much more effectively.

Neck stiffness is not only a health and fitness issue, it is a safety issue too: your peripheral vision is restricted when neck rotation is impeded. Driving and crossing roads are more dangerous when you can't turn your head properly.

The muscles at the side of your neck tend to be the first to lose flexibility and the most likely to create referred pain symptoms in your arms and hands. For this reason, the scalenes on the sides of your neck are known as "the great entrappers."

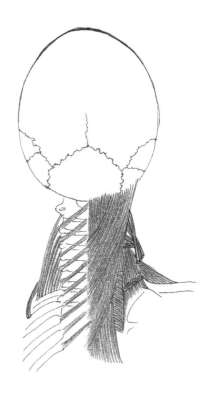

Stiff neck muscles are usually responsible for aches at the back of your head. As we age, the neck can become sensitive to wind and breezes outdoors and to fans and air conditioners indoors. Wearing a light scarf can give surprising relief to this type of neck pain.

Your neck can react very acutely to stress too – when someone is being "a pain in the neck," they often really are. We seem to have a primal instinct to defensively tense the neck muscles, not only to physical threats but to emotional ones too.

Self Massage of the neck can help relieve sinus pain, headaches and insomnia. Care must be taken to avoid direct pressure on the throat and the major blood vessels either side of it. Always apply pressure gradually and Self Massage carefully.

Neck strengthening exercises do not require weights like you would for your biceps. They are done to correct posture and function. Neck stretches should be done every day. Neglecting to do so can result in stiffness that can cause headaches, neck pain and disc degeneration. Think of it as a task like brushing your teeth or getting dressed.

If you have a past neck injury, start with only gentle pressure and exertion. If you experience strong pain, dizziness, lightheadedness, nausea or a headache, stop immediately and see your doctor.

10.1 MUSCLES OF THE NECK AND JAW

The **jaw muscles** can react very acutely to stress, often manifesting as unconscious grinding and tensing. It has long been remarked by bodyworkers that we unconsciously bite down hard in order to stop ourselves from saying how we really feel about others.

Anxiety, anger, intense mental concentration, feeling cold, the over-use of stimulants, gum chewing and dental problems can also produce jaw tension. Jaw tension can prematurely wear away tooth enamel and even cause stress fractures in your teeth.

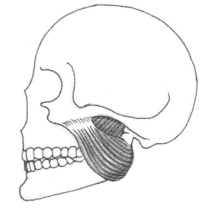

Some of the most severe headaches you will ever experience are the product of untreated jaw tension. They usually occur at the sides of your head. The good news is that Self Massage of your jaw muscles is simple – they are easy to reach and require little pressure.

The **scalenes** are the muscles on the sides of your neck that bend it sideways. When the scalenes get stiff, sideways neck bending gets more difficult. Muscular tension here can cause the nerves that run down to your arms to become irritated, with the result that pain is referred down to your arms. If your elbow becomes inexplicably sore, this may be why.

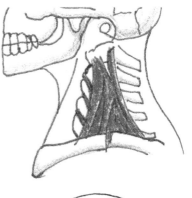

The **sternocleidomastoid** (SCM) muscles at the front of your neck tend to tense sympathetically with tight jaw muscles. They can be Self Massaged, but with great care to avoid pressuring the throat and carotid arteries. This is best achieved by light plucking fingertip movements and pressure – nothing firm. It is good to stretch these muscles too. The SCMs nod your head forward, so they may stiffen if you look down a lot.

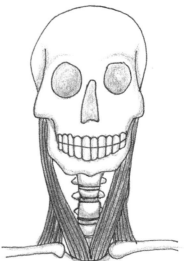

The upper **trapezius** causes your head to move from side to side, and helps you to raise your arms and to shrug. (Other muscles assist this action also – very few movements are controlled by one muscle alone.) The occipital muscles behind your neck enable you to look up. The muscles at the front of your neck nod your head forward and the levator scapulae muscles attached to your shoulder blades rotate your head when you look over your shoulder.) When the upper trapezius is flexed it helps protect your neck.

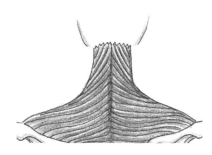

The **levator scapulae** raises your shoulder blades (the scapulae) by pulling them up toward your skull via the attachment points on their inner and upper corners. It helps you to shrug your shoulders and rotate your head to look over your shoulder. If looking right or left feels restricted, your levator scapulae may need massaging and stretching. This muscle usually needs stretching more than strengthening, because it is always working against gravity.

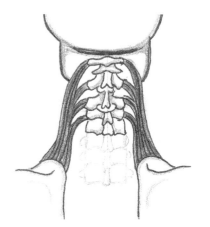

The posterior neck muscles include the **suboccipitals** at the base of the skull and the **splenius** along the back of the neck. Flexing these muscles makes you look directly upward. Computer workers often get shortened posterior neck muscles because of poor work posture (for example, looking too closely at the screen). Often, the back of your neck gets overworked from the use of cell phones and other hand-held devices. Tight posterior neck muscles can make looking up uncomfortable and give you headaches at the back of your head (suboccipital headaches). The suboccipital acupressure points at the base of your skull, when massaged, can calm us down and induce sleep.

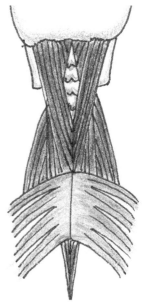

10.2 SELF MASSAGE OF THE NECK AND JAW

N1   Scalene stroke

Sit with one elbow resting on a desk. Use the fingers of that hand to gently palpate the muscles on the opposite side and back of your neck. Feel all around the area searching for the individual muscles and the grooves between them. Some of these muscle strands can be firmer or more sensitive than others. Do this for 3 to 5 minutes, then change hands and do the same to the other side.

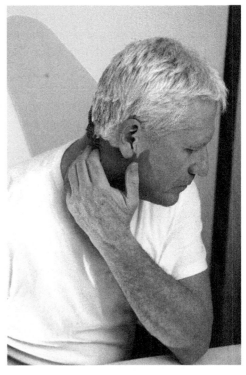

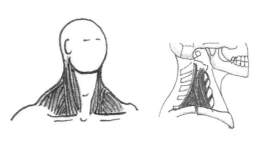

N2   Scalene stroke with tool

Sit in the same position as N1 and place a Thumbsaver on either your index or middle finger. Using it, focus on the tighter muscles you discovered in N1, applying a little more pressure (but not painfully so, as this is supposed to feel good). The Thumbsaver will allow you to apply pressure for longer without tiring your finger and with more pinpoint accuracy than your finger alone. Continue to do this for as long as it feels comfortable and then do the other side of your neck.

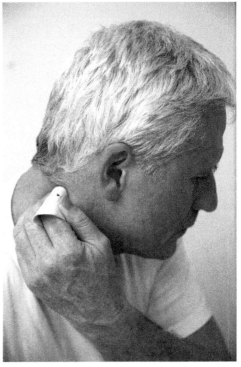

N3 Neck towel roll

Lie either on the floor or on your bed and place a rolled bath towel under your neck. Slowly turn your neck from side to side in a slow gentle rocking motion. After about 6 to 8 turns your neck should start to feel like it rotates more fully. You can do it a few more times if it feels good, but stop anytime it starts to get uncomfortable.

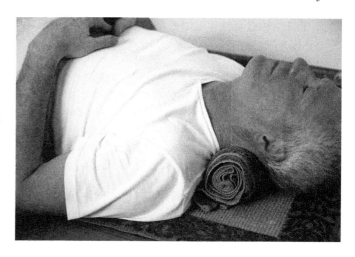

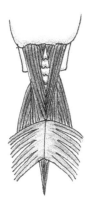

This technique helps maintain the normal curve of your neck. If you often crane your neck forward to look at things, this should help relieve your neck muscles.

N4 Two hand neck rub

Place one hand around the back of your neck and then put your other hand on top of the first to provide support and pressure. By curling your fingertips forward and moving both hands side to side, you can achieve a surprising firmness with little effort. As with the other techniques, it should feel good, not painful. If you lean back in a chair while doing this, you can keep your head comfortably upright.

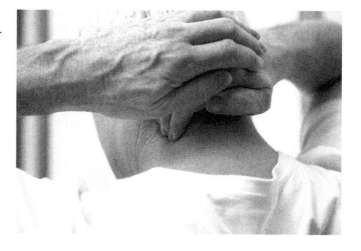

N5 Upward neck slide

Lift an elbow up to head height and reach backward around to the other side of your neck. Apply finger pressure and then **drop your elbow down at the front.** As you do so, your hand will effortlessly move upward in a diagonal direction. You can use a little oil or moisturizer to do this technique so you do not pull any hairs on the back of your neck.

This action uses different muscles than the neck techniques used so far, so you can Self Massage for longer without tiring. If you have a stiff shoulder, however, this may be difficult to execute. Do both sides if you can.

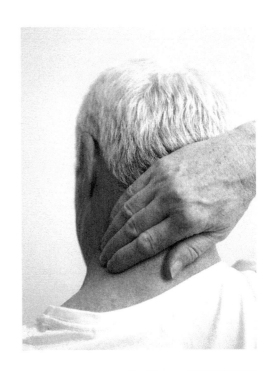

N6 Sideward neck and jaw press

Sit side-on to your desk and rest your elbow on it. Place your hand with the thumb against the neck or jaw, as shown in the photograph. Leave your arm stationary and move your head toward your hand to create a comfortable pressure where your thumb presses the neck or jaw. You can also use your fingers or a Thumbsaver tool to apply pressure.

Pressing below the edge of your skull and cheekbone, you will notice natural indentations. These are pressure points that can help clear your sinuses and relieve headaches.

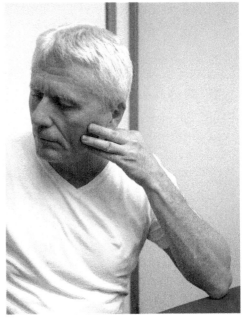

N7 Top shoulder pressure point

With a cushion to kneel on, find an inward pointing wall angle or doorway (that no one will close on your head) and put your shoulder against a tennis ball, as though you are packing into a rugby scrum. Keep ahold of the ball so it does not slip or roll away, and relax the arm on the massaged side. The middle of your upper trapezius muscle is what you are aiming for. This muscle is usually tight on most people and this is an easy way to apply pressure to it. It is one of my favorites. If your knees are bad, it can also be done standing up and bending forward.

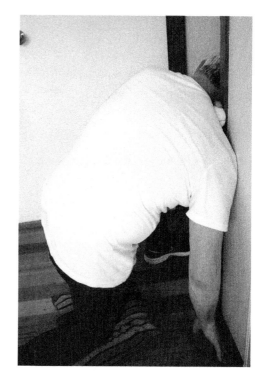

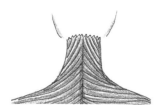

N8 Neck walking stick

Place the "hook" end of a walking stick against your trapezius. With the stick held in an upright position, pull the handle downward. This will work the top of the trapezius muscle.

Alternatively, hold the stick level and pull it away from your body to work the back of the trapezius. In this position, you can also lean backward into a wall for extra pressure (but do it on a brick wall, because it may dent a plaster one).

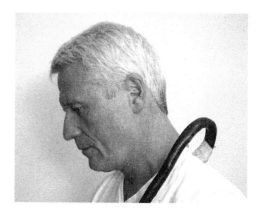

N9 Levered wrist pressure

Sit at a desk and lean on it with your elbow. Place your fingers on your upper trapezius and your jaw over your wrist for leverage. Press down with your fingers, avoiding pressure on your throat.

This technique allows you to Self Massage your upper trapezius muscle without using a stick or a ball.

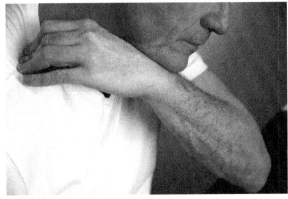

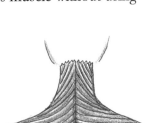

N10 Jaw knuckles

There are a number of things that tighten jaw muscles. Fortunately, these muscles are easy to reach and require little effort for a good massage effect. Move your knuckles around over the muscles to find the hardest spots. Sustain firm but comfortable pressure. After a few minutes your jaw tension should start to ease. Do this exercise regularly if you suffer from jaw tension. Side headaches can also respond well to this technique.

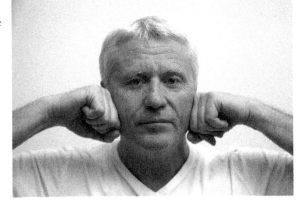

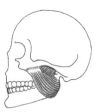

Yawning is a good stretching exercise for your jaw muscles. Jaw tension is a postural problem so you need to regularly remind yourself to hold your jaw loose when you are not talking or eating.

10.3 EXERCISES FOR THE NECK

N11 Side neck flex

Hold your head still and push firmly against the side of your head with the palm of your hand, keeping your neck and head straight. Hold this for at least 30 seconds, and then do the other side.

The muscles on the side of your neck can produce arm pain and weakness as well as neck problems if allowed to stiffen.

Keep your neck straight. Go slowly but firmly.

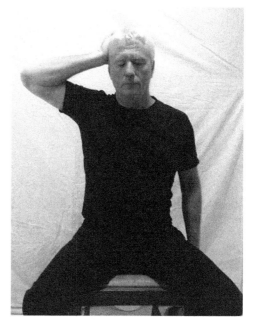

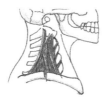

N12 Seated neck side stretch

Sit straight and hold one side of your chair. With your other hand, **gently** and **slowly** stretch your neck sideways. Keep your neck relaxed and your back straight. Hold the stretch for 20 seconds, then change hands and do the other side.

Holding your shoulder down helps to maximize this stretch. The other hand is not pulling the head sideways so much as creating a traction weight.

This is a good upper trapezius and scalene stretch. Your upper trapezius is a shoulder muscle as well as a neck muscle. It needs to be stretched often, as there are many people who are chronically tight in these muscles.

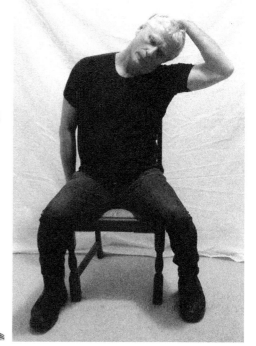

N13 Diagonal neck stretch

When neck rotation and shrugging of the shoulders feels impeded, it could be the result of stiffness in the **levator scapulae**. The curved motion of the levator scapulae rotates your head, so this exercise can ease stiff neck rotation.

Sit with a straight back and hold the back corner of your chair. Lean your head diagonally forward at about 45 degrees. Use your other hand to gently assist the stretch of the levator scapulae.
Maintain this position for 30 to 60 seconds. Then do the other side. **Go gently**. If this hurts, stop immediately.

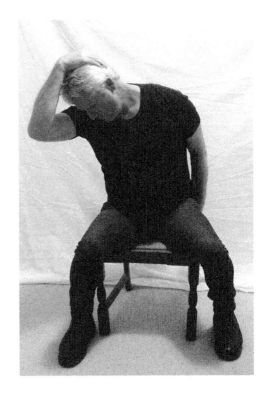

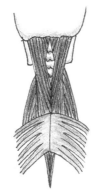

N14 Back of neck flex

Sit straight on a chair and interlock your fingers behind your head. Gently but firmly push your head backward into your hands for 20 seconds.

Keep your neck and head straight so you are upright and pushing back against your hands. This exercise will help correct your posture and stretch the muscles on the back and side of your neck, which get fatigued and tighten with sedentary jobs. It is good for relief of pain at the back of your neck after you have been craning your neck forward (like when you look down to write a text message).

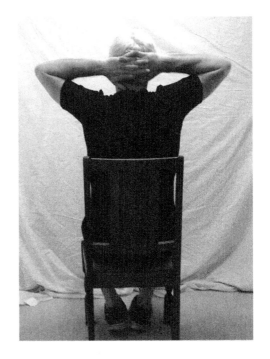

70

11 UPPER BODY

The muscles on the front and back of your upper body power your shoulders, upper arms, upper back and your breathing. Some upper body muscles extend up to the neck and others downward to the lower body.

From age 40 onward, shoulder problems such as frozen shoulder (adhesive capsulitis) and fibromyalgia become more common. Self Massage can be of assistance in alleviating these conditions and can help make muscles exercise-ready. If you have been neglecting to stretch these muscles and allowed them to lose their normal flexibility, the Self Massage techniques in this chapter can not only help you restore movement but also help prevent muscle and joint injury.

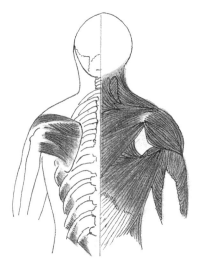

The muscles in this part of your body are used when you breathe, so you may also experience an easier breathing sensation through Self Massaging.

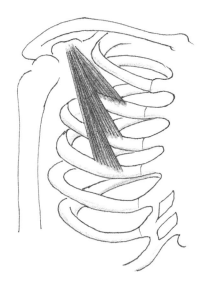

There are seven layers of muscle in your back. The sensations you will experience as you Self Massage are the result of the pressure used, the direction of pressure, and progressive loosening through the layers of muscle.

It is easy to forget what it is like to feel normal, so you may not even notice how much you have tightened up until you attempt to loosen these muscles.

If you have ever had a shoulder dislocation, extra caution is required with exercises that raise your arms above your head or behind your back. It is best to ask the advice of your doctor or physiotherapist about which exercises in this book are suitable for you, especially if your shoulder dislocation is still unstable.

As previously mentioned in this book, any Self Massage technique that gives you sharp pain should be avoided. These techniques should feel good, not bad.

11.1 MUSCLES OF THE UPPER BODY

The **pectorals** and **anterior deltoids** in your chest and shoulders enable you to reach forward and across the front of your upper body. Whenever you hug someone or reach over your shoulder for a seatbelt, for example, you engage these muscles. They can tighten and interfere with correct upright posture, which in turn causes neck and upper back pain. Tight pectorals can also restrict normal breathing.

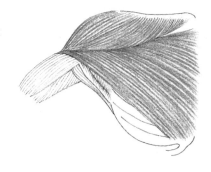

The **infraspinatus, teres minor** and **teres major** over your shoulder blades enable you to raise your arms in front of your body to do things like opening doors, using keyboards and cooking. They are very busy muscles and are chronically tight on computer workers. Self Massaging them is highly recommended if you have this type of job. For best results, it is good to stretch these muscles after Self Massaging them.

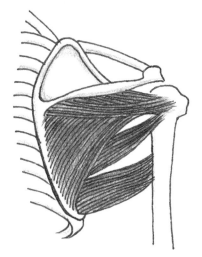

The **rhomboids** draw your shoulder blades back and up. Most of us get stiff and weak in these important muscles. The techniques in this chapter are very useful in loosening them. It is usually easier to Self Massage these muscles straight up and down rather than sideways.

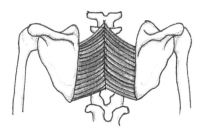

When rhomboids are weak, your shoulders slump forward. Good rhomboid tone is important for good posture and allows you to breathe more easily. Rowing exercises strengthen the rhomboids – rowers usually have nice upright postures.

The **deltoids** cover your shoulders and get their name from their triangular shape. They help move your arms upward, outward and backward. Big deltoids make your shoulders look wider. Whenever you lift anything up or swim, you engage these muscles.

Self Massaging and stretching these muscles helps you to maintain your normal reach and shoulder flexibility. If you strengthen your deltoids with the right exercises, your posture can benefit as well as your lifting ability.

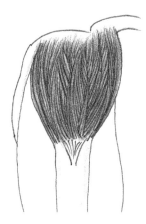

Your **latissimus dorsi** ("lats") enable you to climb, swim, row, lift heavy things off high shelves, and raise and lower yourself onto and off armchairs.

When your lats are exercised regularly, they give your back the classic "V-shaped" look that tapers down toward your waist. Toned lats look good on men and women alike. Swimmers have good lats.

In the illustration at right, you can see why your lats have the potential to sculpt the shape of your body, with the muscle being attached to your ribs, upper arms and spine.

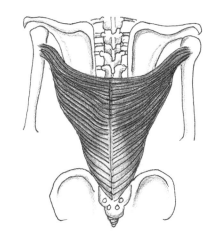

The upper **trapezius** (view from front shown at right) moves your head sideways and raises your shoulders. It helps protect your neck if it is suddenly bent sideways, and holds your head straight when flexed evenly on both sides. The trapezius tends to react strongly to stress, so it needs frequent massage and stretching for comfort and good posture.

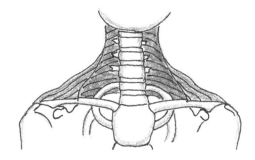

11.2 SELF MASSAGE OF THE UPPER BODY

S1   Chest finger press

Apply simple downward pressure with the fingertips to the front of your chest (pectorals). Search for the tender pressure points and the strands of muscle fiber that surround them. It can be quite surprising how little pressure it takes to be aware of sensitivity in these muscles. The areas of greatest sensitivity usually require the most Self Massage. A small massage tool can be used for this too.

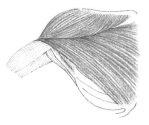

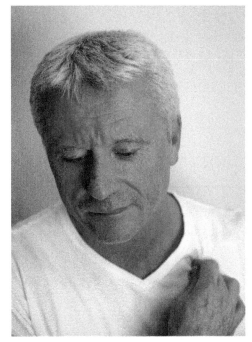

S2   Shoulder wall roll

This technique applies stronger pressure to the pectorals. Turn your body at an angle toward a wall and place a tennis ball between your chest and the wall. Work the muscle from side to side and in a circular fashion. Initiate movement from your hips, using a wide stance and with even weight on both feet for good balance. The further your feet are from the wall, the stronger the pressure will be.

Try doing this for a few minutes to start with.

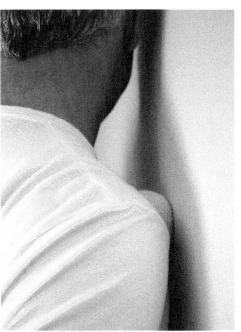

S3   Shoulder blade wall roll

Stand with your feet a shoulder's width apart and turn your back at an angle to a wall. Position a tennis ball (or a ball that is slightly softer) between your shoulder blade and the wall, and use a circular motion to Self Massage the muscles over the shoulder blade.

These muscles can become very sensitive through activities that take your arm through short repetitious movements, such as using a computer mouse (I refer to this as mouse shoulder). Office workers should do this technique every day.

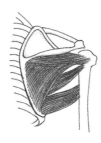

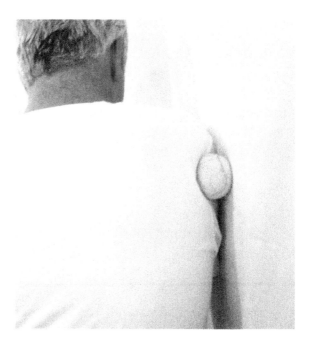

S4   Upper back wall roll

Turn your back at 45 degrees to a wall and position a tennis ball between your spine and shoulder blade. Lean in toward the wall to apply pressure and slowly move your body up and down.

The rhomboids are the target muscles in this technique. They can feel surprisingly sensitive, so go easy to start with. This technique works best when you can fully relax into the pressure, so apply less pressure if you cannot relax.

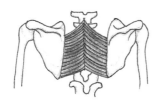

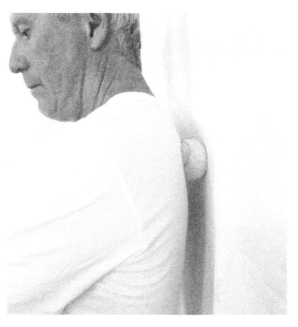

S5 Two ball wall roll

For this technique, position two tennis balls between a wall and your upper back. The balls should be of equal hardness, one on each side of your spine, and at the same level. Work the balls up and down by bending and straightening your knees. As always, relax into the technique and work within your pressure tolerances. Stand with even weight on both feet.

You can put the balls into a sock together if you find them hard to control separately.

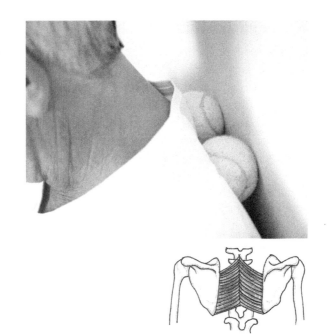

S6 Upper back corner slide

Lean backward into a doorway or wall angle so you can feel contact on the band of muscle between your spine and shoulder blade. Stand with even weight on both feet and move your body slowly from side to side. If the edge feels too sharp, wear an extra layer of clothing or reduce the force by moving your feet closer to the wall.

This is a handy technique to loosen tight upper back muscles when you have no massage tools. It can help loosen tight rowing muscles.

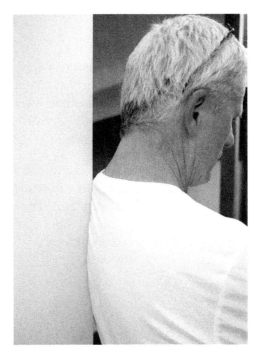

S7 Deltoid wall roll

Stand side-on to a wall and use a tennis ball in an up and down motion to apply pressure to the deltoid muscle group. Work within your comfort zone and do both sides.

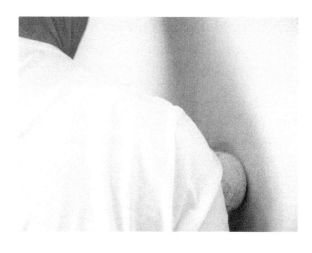

If it feels a little tricky to stop the ball slipping out, steady the sides of the ball with your other hand, or use a smaller ball. Stand straight.

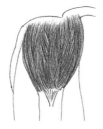

S8 Deltoid cross grip

Reach across your chest and grip into the groove in the deltoid muscle, rolling your fingertips sideways across the muscles. Do both sides.

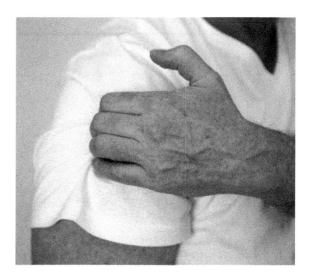

You don't need a ball or a wall for this Self Massage technique, just a reasonably firm grip that you move from side to side. It works best when the massaged arm is dangling completely relaxed by your side. A massage tool can be utilized for this technique too.

Like **S7 Deltoid wall roll**, this technique can help relieve the symptoms of frozen shoulder. You can do this anywhere and anytime, sitting or standing.

S9 Shoulder corner press

You can use either a doorway or an internal wall angle for this exercise. Place your near foot back and your opposite foot forward, and press your shoulder against the wall so you can feel your shoulder blade sliding backward over your ribs. Turn your head away from the wall, and move your weight to your front foot as you ease forward.

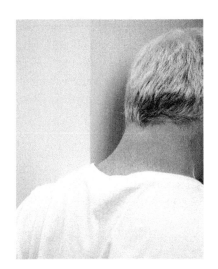

This technique is as much a stretch as it is Self Massage. This is a great technique to practice after exercising your chest and shoulder muscles, or for opening your chest up after a long day at the computer.

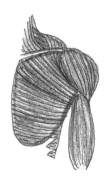

S10 Chest plunger press

Stick your sink plunger to the wall and hold its shaft so its end is located directly in the groove between the chest and shoulder muscles. Place one foot forward and the other back and gradually lean forward until you feel a pleasant tension relief that opens your chest up. **Do not let go of the plunger until you finish.**

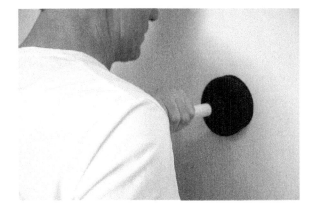

Wrap some cloth tape around the end of the plunger for extra comfort if you wish.

11.3 EXERCISES FOR THE UPPER BODY

Your shoulders are easily the most mobile large joints in your body, enabled by an open socket and a complex muscle structure. This happens somewhat at the expense of the stability of the shoulder joint, which is dislocated much more easily and often than our other large joints.

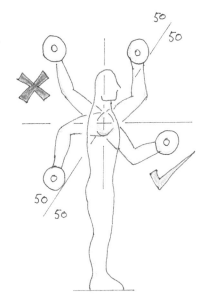

Your shoulders work much more efficiently when you are using your arms in front of your body, at and below the height of the shoulders. Reaching upward and behind are movements that the shoulders are not nearly as strong, efficient or stable at.

For this reason, resistance exercises that push weights above the head and behind the body are not recommended in this book. There are safer and more effective ways to strengthen your arm and upper body muscles.

The chest and upper back muscles are grouped together with the shoulder muscles in this chapter because of their proximity to and synergy with each other.

When exercising these muscles, always be attentive to your form (posture). This applies regardless of whether you are engaged in cardio, stretching or resistance exercise. Whether you are lifting a box at work, your child at home or weights in a gym, the safe way to do it is always the same: with a straight back, upright head, and your legs doing most of the work. Good form is not just about the exercise itself – it is also about getting into the right position before you start.

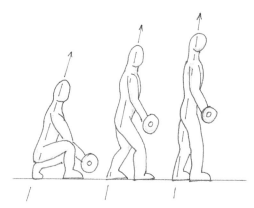

Also, always make sure to move in one plane of motion at a time: do not bend and twist as you lift.

Good balance is important for all upper body exercise. Be sure to exercise right and left sides evenly, and to exercise the upper body muscles on the front and back of your body evenly for good posture. A strong upper back opens your chest, which helps your breathing and makes you look taller and more confident.

S11 Wall push-up

Face into a corner with your feet a shoulder's width apart, and push into and away from the corner. The further your feet are from the wall, the more strenuous this exercise becomes.

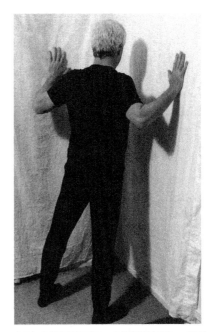

> Push-ups and bench press are exercises that have a reputation for increasing shoulder, chest and upper arm strength. This is the easiest push-up to do. When the wall push-up gets easy to do and you want something a little harder, go on to knee push-ups. When 30 of those becomes easy, move onto standard push-ups.

S12 Knee push-up

Lie face down with your hands pressing against the floor in front of your shoulders. Bend your knees so your feet are up, then fully extend your arms into the knee push-up position, as shown at right. Then steadily lower your body almost to the floor, and repeat. Do not rush this exercise.

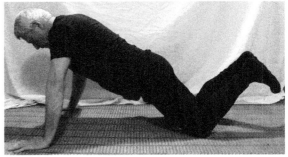

This is the easiest floor push-up. Since women usually have less upper body strength than men, they may not need any of the more strenuous push-ups below.

S13 Standard push-up

Standard push-ups are done with legs extended straight and toes on the floor. Keep your body and legs in a straight line as you raise your body to the position shown at right, and then steadily lower it almost completely to the floor. Keep this action smooth and unhurried.

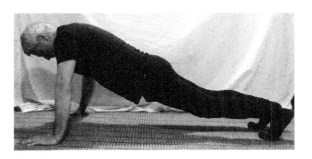

S14 Rolling push-up

If the standard push-up starts to feel easy and you can do 30 or more without much effort, it could be time to increase the degree of difficulty in order to get stronger and avoid repetitive strain injury.

Rolling push-ups are a popular martial arts exercise. They are not only harder to do than standard push-ups, but also engage a greater number of muscles, such as your lats and your thigh muscles. They are executed in a more natural circular motion than the standard up-and-down push-up.

Exercising your lats with rolling pushups not only strengthens and enlarges the shoulders and chest, it also gives that "V" shape that strong swimmers get, flattering to both the male and female form.

Start in the normal push-up position with your body straight and arms fully extended.

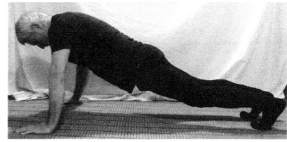

Raise your butt and push it backward in a steady controlled movement, until it is above your knees. Move your body backward until your arms are fully extended.

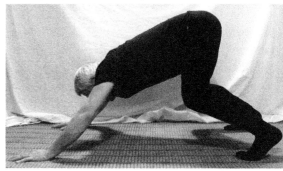

Lower your body and keep your elbows level with your shoulders as you move forward. The floor passes just beneath your face, as though you are slowly swooping down like a bird. Then return to the starting position.

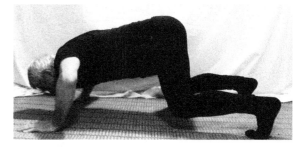

S15 Bench press

Starting with weights that you are easily able to pick up, lock them evenly onto the bar. Lie on your back under the bar and lower the bar to your chest, then raise it again. Grip completely around the bar and keep your back flat to the bench. The bench press exercises the arms, shoulders and chest in a similar manner to push-ups.

The bench press is a very popular gym exercise. It can be effective but also dangerous. If your strength fails during a push-up, you fall a short distance; with a failed bench press, you can crush your windpipe. If there is one exercise for which spotting with a partner is **essential**, it is this one.

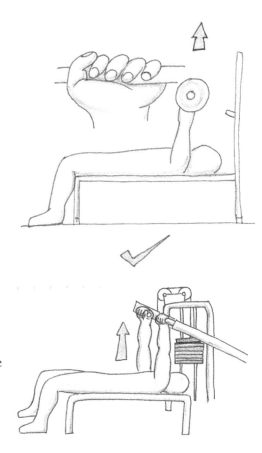

S16 Machine bench press

Machine bench press is the same as bench press with the added safety that the weight cannot fall onto your chest or throat. Check that you can push the weight up with fully extended arms. Raise and lower the weight until you start to tire.

While safer to use, lifting machines are not as time efficient as a free weight bench press, because synergizing and stabilizing muscles are not used as much.

S17 Lateral shoulder press

Lateral shoulder press is like a bench press, except that you are pushing forward rather than upward. Keep your back and neck straight as you fully extend into the lift. Repeat this motion until you start to tire.

> S11 to S17 are all different methods of strengthening your upper arms, shoulders and chest. Be sure to mix these exercises with upper back rowing type exercises.

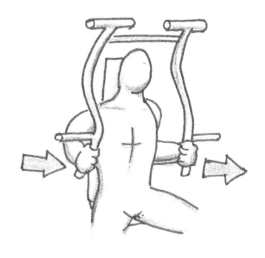

S18 Backward arm stretch

Place one foot forward and the other back in a wide stance, with the back foot nearest the wall. Place the palm of the near hand up on the wall behind you, as shown at right. With your arm locked straight, lean in toward the wall while turning your head away from the wall. Breathe out as you stretch. Maintain this position for at least 20 seconds, then do the other side.

When done properly, this stretch is very effective in stretching your chest and shoulder muscles, giving you relief from muscle tension and helping to straighten your posture. It can also give your calf, thigh, and hip flexor muscles relief.

Most of us have jobs where we are constantly reaching forward to do things – using tools, typing, cooking, digging, driving, packing and looking after kids. These tasks can all tighten up our shoulders. This stretch can help.

If your shoulder dislocates easily, don't do this stretch.

Whatever is flexed also needs to be stretched. Failure to stretch your anterior deltoids (front of your shoulder) and pectorals (chest muscles) will eventually cause your shoulders to feel tight and appear hunched forward.

Backward arm stretch is a good multiple muscle stretch. Exercises such as this are a good warm-down for the resistance exercises in this chapter.

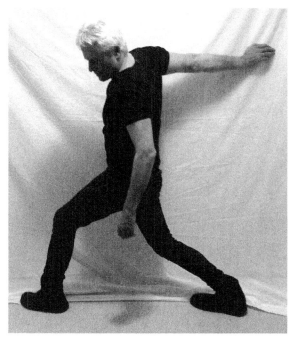

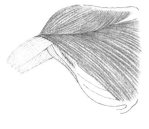

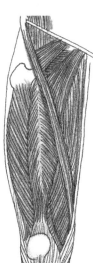

S19 Backward ball stretch

Swiss Balls are very useful in a variety of exercises. They can be purchased for a much lower cost in department stores now than they were previously priced in sports stores. They come in different sizes, so observe the manufacturer's recommendation for your height and weight.

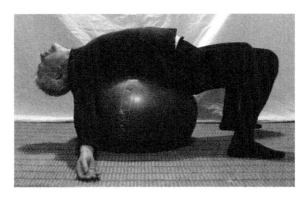

In this shoulder and chest stretch, drape your body backward on the ball and let your arms hang over the sides. Slowly move your upper and mid back over the ball. Your arms will change position as you do so and you will feel your chest and shoulder muscles stretch differently each time you change position. For best results, move slowly, pause, and relax into any stretch that feels good.

When done properly, this stretch should not hurt. If you feel any pain or dizziness, do not persist.

Be attentive to your balance. Keeping your feet a shoulder's width apart will help stabilize any unintended sideways movement. Ensure that there are no hard or sharp objects in your general vicinity that you might fall onto.

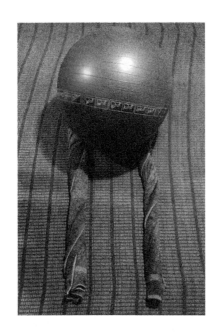

If your balance is a bit wobbly, roll a pair of towels to prevent the ball moving sideways, as shown at right.

If you have recently sustained a back injury, do not attempt this exercise.

S20 Corner shoulder stretch

Face into a corner with your hands on the walls at neck height and your feet a shoulder's width apart. Lean forward while pressing against the walls. Hold the stretch for 20 to 30 seconds. When you finish, you should feel like your chest is open and your spine is upright.

This exercise looks very similar to **S11 Wall push-up**, but you are letting yourself drop into the corner in order to stretch the chest and the front of the shoulders.

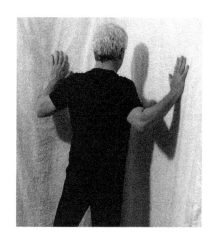

S21 Open chest stretch

Grasp your left wrist with your right hand behind your back. Stand straight and pull your wrists backward as far as you can in a smooth motion. Exhale while making this movement. As with all other stretches, **do not** do this with jerking or bouncing movements, but keep the motion smooth and controlled. Hold the stretch and relax into it for 20 to 30 seconds as you slowly exhale. Then change your grip to the other side and repeat.

This stretch can be done as often as you feel the need to, throughout the day or night. It is a dual exercise: it strengthens the upper back and also stretches the chest and shoulders.

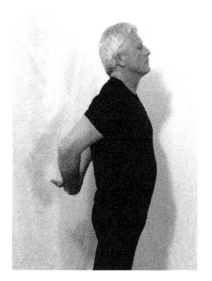

The rhomboid muscles are the ones most specifically strengthened with this exercise. Most of us have weak rhomboids because we rarely use them during the course of the average working day. This is partly why so many of us slouch forward so much of the time. Weak rhomboids can produce upper back and neck pain.

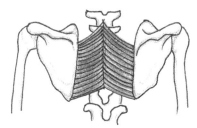

S22 Rowing machine

The rowing machine strengthens the upper arms, thighs, shoulders and back. Keep your back straight through the whole action as you bend and straighten your knees.

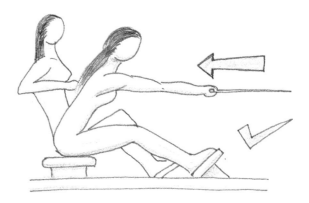

Rowing machines have long been a popular whole body exerciser. Be careful when using this apparatus that you **do not** throw yourself too far back and **hyperextend** your lower back like an Olympic rower does.

Done with low intensity this is cardio and with high intensity it is strength training. Check the tension on the machine before you begin.

S23 Upper back band flex

Stand straight and grasp the ends of a Thera-Band that matches your strength. Pull the ends of the Thera-Band out sideways to fully extend your arms. You should feel the rhomboids between your shoulder blades working. Hold for 5 seconds and repeat until you start to tire.

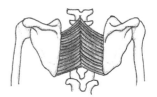

This exercise feels great when you have been stuck behind a computer all day. If one Thera-Band doesn't provide enough resistance, use two.

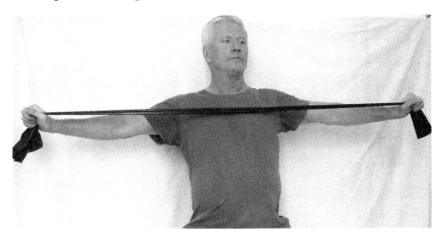

S24 Isolateral row

The **isolateral row** is a strengthening exercise for your upper back and arms. It works your upper back in a lateral plane of motion and allows you to keep your spine straight.

This exercise is like a rowing machine except that you are sitting higher and isolating the muscles of the upper body. If you have a sore lower back, this is a safer exercise than the rowing machine.

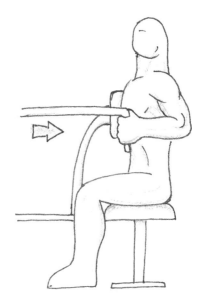

S25 Rotated body stretch

Place one foot well in front of the other and extend the arm on the side of the rear foot out in front of you. Place the wrist of the other hand behind its elbow and slowly twist sideways until you are at full rotation, as shown at right. **Do not twist rapidly or use short jerking movements**. Hold this position for 20 seconds as you breathe out, then do the other side.

If you rotate from your hips, you should feel the stretch from your spine across your upper back right up to your elbow. This also stretches your groin, hip flexors and calves. Stand near a wall in case you over-balance.

This is a good warm-down stretch after exercising your upper back.

Do not force this exercise. If you have a current lower back injury, avoid any exercise that produces sharp pain.

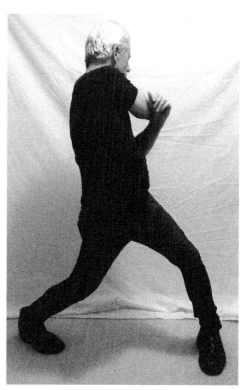

S26 Pec deck

The **Pec Deck** is specifically made to increase chest muscle (pectorals) size and strength. Begin with your hands just **forward** of your shoulders and move your arms evenly through the full movement. If you cannot smoothly control the movement, reduce the load. Keep an upright posture and do not lean forward into it. **If you twinge or struggle, stop immediately**.

It is important to keep your hands in front of your shoulders at all times.

A good warm-down after this exercise is stretching exercises like **S18 Backward arm stretch**.

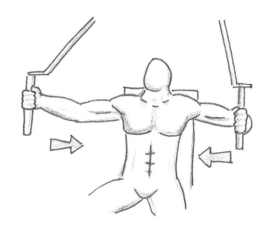

S27 Chest band flex

Tie one end of a Thera-Band around something stable at a suitable height, such as a doorknob. Stand **side-on** to where the Thera-Band is fastened. Pull the loose end of the Thera-Band across your chest, in a similar motion to reaching for the seat belt in a car. (Next time you reach across your chest for a seat belt, place your other hand over your chest muscle. You will feel it tense up as you do so.) This is a direct way to strengthen and enlarge your chest muscles. You can use two bands if you feel you need more resistance.

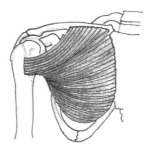

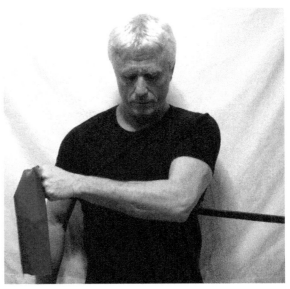

S28 Lat pull-down

The lat pull-down is performed in the seated position. You should feel the sides of your shoulders and upper back doing the work as you pull the handles directly downward to chest height. Most machines will have a pad that holds your thighs down.

It is important to keep your spine straight throughout the whole motion to ensure that you do not hyperextend your spine backward. **Pull down, not back**.

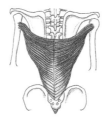

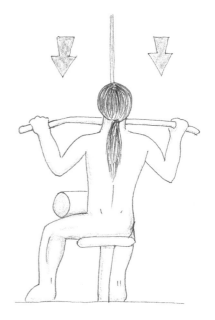

Shown above is the correct form (posture) of lat pull-down. The method shown at right, where the bar is pulled down behind your head, is **not correct**. The muscles of the shoulders fight against one another and the neck is cocked forward, which distorts the shape of your spine and compromises its strength.

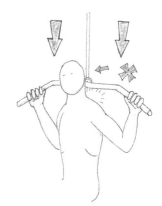

Doing lat pull-downs this way is a common error, and while you may get away with doing it this way for a while, it will eventually cause you harm.

S29 The child stretch

From your hands and knees, move your body backward to lower your butt onto your heels while leaving your palms on the floor. Your arms will stretch out in front of you as you stretch your shoulder muscles. Hold for at least 20 seconds. If your knees are not the best, you can kneel on a thin cushion or reach up and lean against a wall in a similar fashion. **If your shoulders dislocate easily, avoid this stretch**.

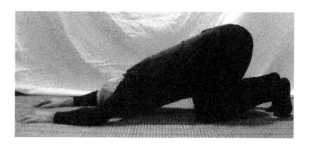

S30 Chin-ups

Firmly grasp the bar and steadily raise your body until your chin is level with the bar. Then steadily lower yourself again until your upper arms are below your elbows, and repeat.

If you cannot lift your whole body weight, start out by keeping your feet on the floor and gradually taking more weight with your hands and less through your feet.

Chin-ups (also known as pull-ups) strengthen your shoulders, arms, abs and back. Lift yourself so that the bar is in front of your face, not behind your neck. Similarly to lat pull-downs, placing the bar behind your head places unnecessary stress on the neck and shoulders. Keep your back straight throughout the exercise.

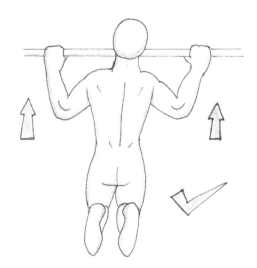

A chin-up bar that is too thin might hurt your hands, while a bar that is too thick is hard to grip properly. Purpose-made chin-up bars such as those pictured at right are easy to find and use. The upper two can be supported by older style upper architraves and are easily lifted into place, while the third requires small metal cups to be screwed into the doorway. Please ensure that the timber where the bar is fitted is in good condition and be sure that the manufacturer's recommended weight capacity is not exceeded by your own bodyweight.

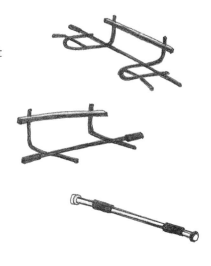

You can also find stronger and heavier chin-up bars that can be screwed into walls. These are similar to those you will find in gymnasiums. Many parks now have exercise stations with chin-up bars.

If you choose to improvise with a non-purpose-made horizontal bar, make sure that it will properly support your body weight. Dangling from an overhead drainpipe that gives way can really get you into trouble.

S31 Lat wall stretch

Raise your upper arm so your elbow is above your head, and place a ball between the thick uppermost part of your shoulder and the wall. Position your feet so that the foot closest to the wall is set back and the other foot is forward. Lean sideways against the wall, then bend and straighten your knees to move the ball along your lats and triceps.

This technique also stretches your lats as you massage them. In the Advanced Self Massage chapter you will find a firmer method of working your lats, but try this one first.

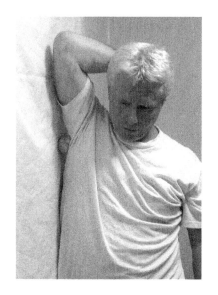

S32 Shrugs

The aptly named **Shrugs** are best executed with dumbbells by your sides rather than with a barbell in front of you, because it is easier to keep your back straight. Stand with your feet a shoulder's width apart and shrug your shoulders up and down while firmly grasping the dumbbells. Heavy weights are not necessary for this exercise to be effective.

Shrugs can also be done with Thera-Bands. Stand with a band under the outer edge of each foot and hold the other end of each band in your hands as you shrug your shoulders.

Do not do shrugs if you have a neck injury or soreness.

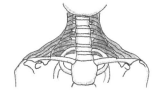

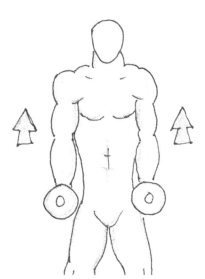

11.4 RISKY UPPER BODY EXERCISES

Upright row is a popular upper back exercise that I wish was **not** popular for the following reasons. First, upright row cannot be performed without leaning forward from your lower back, which is bad for your lower spinal discs. Second, the upper trapezius gets overworked from the lifting motion. The upright row can stiffen your neck and lower back.

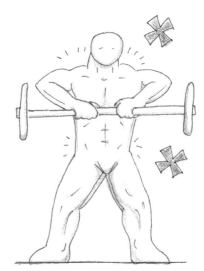

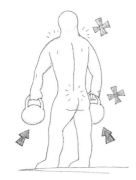

Whether with a bar or kettle bells, you should avoid this exercise unless you play contact sport or participate in competitive weightlifting.

The **shoulder press** has an even greater potential for injury than the upright row. Regardless of whether you attempt shoulder press with free weights or a lifting machine, there are no benefits from this exercise that cannot be achieved with safer methods. If you have a slender build with round shoulders, this applies even more. This is not a comfortable exercise at the best of times and in most gyms I have been to, the shoulder press machines lay dormant most of the time. When this lift goes wrong it goes **really** wrong. **Incline press** is not good for your shoulders either. Shoulder press can also exacerbate spondylolisthesis in your back.

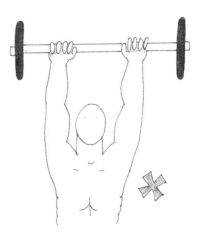

This is a **spondylolisthesis**. It is a spinal problem that not only middle aged and elderly people get, but even some teenagers. It can be excruciating painful. You can clearly see here the misalignment between the bones in the lower back. Lifting weights and violent movements of the spine such as in gymnastics can cause and/or worsen this condition. **Keeping your back straight when you lift** is your best defense against lifting injuries. Lifting weight above your head can worsen a disc injury or weakness through hyperextension of the lower back.

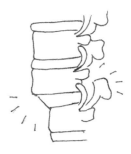

12 ARMS & HANDS

It is easy to take a perfectly functioning pair of arms and hands for granted. It is not until something goes wrong with these ingenious biological tools that we realize how important they are and how little independence we have without them.

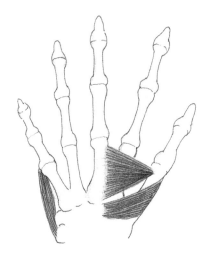

The techniques and exercises in this chapter can help you avoid and recover from common complaints such as Tennis Elbow, Carpal Tunnel Syndrome and Golfer's Elbow.

Our hands take a beating from using tools, cleaning, washing, cooking, gardening, punching, climbing, sailing, using keyboards, and lifting. No other part of our body shows how hard we work. You may consider yourself free of any arm or hand problem at all, only to find after doing some Self Massage that your arms suddenly feel lighter and more flexible than they have for years.

Our lower arms are the engines of our hands, as the hands themselves have little muscle within them. When we grasp, squeeze and climb, it is the muscles beneath our forearms that enable this. When we cock our wrists back to write, type and hit backhanders, it is the muscles on the top of our forearms doing the work.

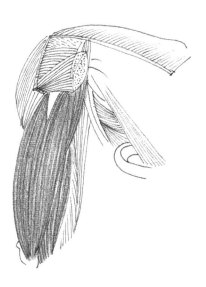

The more powerful muscles of the upper arm are for pushing, pulling, lifting, punching, rowing, chopping and carrying. Sport can really knock elbows and shoulders around – throwing, rowing, playing racquet sports, martial arts and football are tough on your arms. Working with heavy tools and materials are common elbow stressors.

People rarely book themselves in for an arm and hand massage, but they are always surprised by how good they feel after I spend a few minutes massaging their arms.

This chapter shows you how you can do it for yourself.

12.1 MUSCLES OF THE ARMS AND HANDS

The **triceps** straighten the elbow. Whenever you push your arms forward, these muscles engage. If you like doing push-ups, bench presses, martial arts, swimming or boxing, you will use these muscles extensively.

Strong triceps can help cushion your landing if you fall forward. It is not only slower reflexes that makes falling over more dangerous for the elderly – weak arms are less able to absorb the shock from falling.

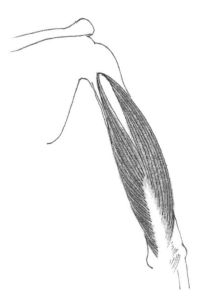

Your **biceps** bend your elbow – the opposite action of the triceps. These two muscle groups have an *agonist/antagonist* relationship. As mentioned in the Strength Training chapter, it is beneficial for your joints (in this case the elbow) to have strength symmetry between the agonists and antagonists.

Your biceps are used when you hug and when you lift objects toward your chest. If you use free weights, you will use your biceps a lot, so give them plenty of Self Massage if you do. A good pair of guns stretching your short-sleeved shirt can look impressive. Just remember to be kind to your elbows and lower back when training.

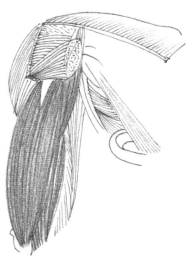

Your **brachioradialis** is engaged when you turn your hands sideways and lift from your elbows – for example, when picking a child up under their arms. There are a lot of mothers of small children with aching brachioradialii. Nurses use these muscles frequently when helping patients to sit and stand up. The use of walking sticks and crutches requires these muscles too. The brachioradialis assists elbow flexion. If you want to get strong looking forearms, brachioradialis exercises can help achieve this.

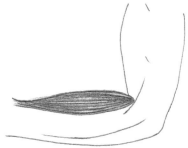

Your **wrist flexors** are the muscles that enable your hands to grasp objects, to make a fist and to bend the wrist forward. Workers in manual occupations often get strong wrist flexors, as do swimmers, bakers and masseurs. Picking up weights in a gym also gives wrist flexors a lot to do. When these muscles are overworked, they can cause weakness, pain and tingling in your hand.

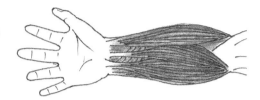

Your **wrist extensors** are opposite to your wrist flexors and are on the back of the forearm. The wrist extensors contract when you straighten your fingers or bend your wrist backward. Hitting back-handers, playing a piano, riding a motorbike, using keyboards and sail boarding all engage your wrist extensors. These muscles are used for fine motor skills like writing, embroidery and needlework.

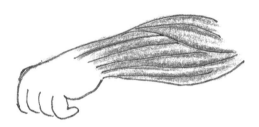

The **thenar** muscles of the hand are for precision movements of the fingers and thumb. Your hands need to be kept supple and flexible as well as strong, because as we age our hands tend to stiffen and weaken. Stretching exercises for the hands are therefore very important – to lose dexterity is to lose fine motor skills and independence. If you make strenuous use of your hands, you also need to massage them.

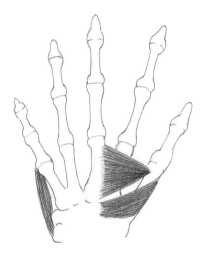

Stress, liver disease, neurological disorders and alcoholism can all affect fine muscle control in your hands.

There is more information about hand Self Massage in the Self-Acupressure & Shiatsu and Reflexology chapters in Part III of this book.

12.2 SELF MASSAGE OF THE ARMS AND HANDS

A1 Cross triceps rub

Reach across your chest and hook your hand around the back of your upper arm. Move your hand backward and forward across your triceps. You don't need much force to do this. Make sure that you Self Massage both sides of the elbow. You may be surprised at the sensitivity of these muscles.

Elbows can stiffen if using weights, so keeping these muscles massaged will help prevent injury and muscle fatigue.

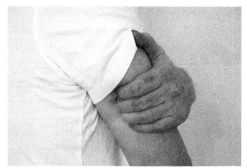

A2 Fist triceps rub

Reach across your chest, make a fist, and hold it against your ribs. Then press your triceps down against your knuckles. Without moving the fist, move your upper arm against it while feeling for the natural grooves in the muscle. Vary the angle of your fist and your upper arm movement to Self Massage the whole of the triceps, while keeping your back straight. You might be surprised at how some muscle strands will feel, even though you didn't even notice they were tight. I use this technique often, and my arms always feel better for it.

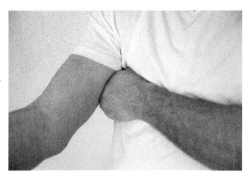

A3 Biceps fist rub

Reach across your chest and use your fist to rub along the other biceps. You won't need to use much pressure to really feel those muscles being worked.

The lower biceps just above the elbow can get particularly sensitive, and massaging it can relieve elbow stiffness.

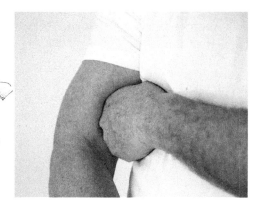

A4 Radialis rub

Rest an arm on a cushion on your lap or on a desk
beside you. Use the other fist to Self Massage the
brachioradialis, using a motion like ironing a shirt.
Self Massage of the forearms is good for your
elbows, wrists and hands.

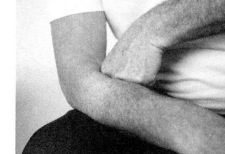

A5 Elbow knuckle

Reach across the front of your lower chest, make a
fist, and hold it against the side of your ribs. Press
the wrist flexors of the other arm against your
stationary knuckles and move the underside of your
forearm against them. As you do so, feel for the
grooves in your muscles. Rock climbers, riders,
baseball players, swimmers, weightlifters and tennis
players all need to take good care of these muscles.
You may be surprised at how effective and easy this
technique is.

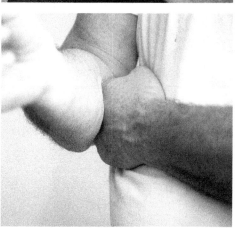

A6 Ball elbow

Stand at approximately 45 degrees to a wall, with your arm
against your side and elbow bent. Place a tennis ball
between the back of your forearm and the wall. Rotate
your body back and forth from your
hips to roll the ball along the wrist
flexors, working from your wrist to
your elbow. Keep your arm relaxed –
the pressure is provided by your
body pressing your arm onto the ball.

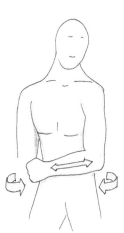

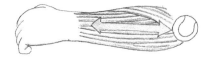

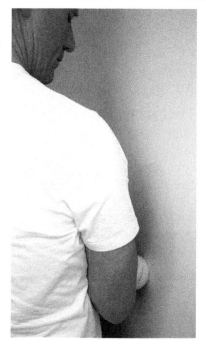

A7 Elbow ratchet rub

Sit diagonally to your desk. Lean on it with your elbow and rest your chin on your upward-facing palm. Grasp around your lower arm with your fingertips hooking in toward your wrist extensors, and move your active massaging arm in a back and forth ratchet-like motion. This is a cross-fiber technique that firmly flicks across the muscle. It works across the muscles whereas **A6 Ball elbow** works along them, so you should do them both.

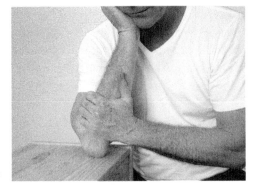

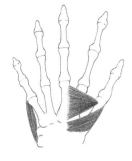

A8 Thumb press

The **thenar** muscles, which move your thumbs, are the busiest muscles in your hands. Use the thumb and index finger of one hand in a pincer-like movement to Self Massage the thenar muscles of the other. If you want extra pressure, use a small massage tool. Give equal attention to the thenar muscles on your palm at the base of your thumb and those between your thumb and index finger.

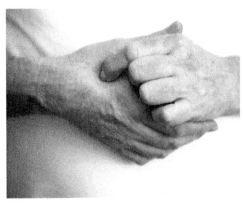

A9 Pinky knuckle

The **hypothenar** muscles are located on the opposite side of your hand to the thenar muscles, below your little finger. Self Massage them by rubbing them against the knuckles of your other hand.

The hypothenar muscles help spread your fingers apart. Artists, craftsmen, surgeons and anyone engaged in fine detail work often use these muscles when the little finger acts as a steady support for the weight of the hand.

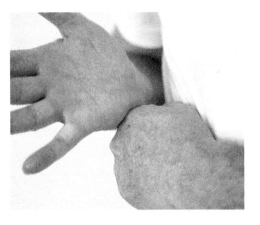

12.3 EXERCISES FOR THE ARMS AND HANDS

A10 Kickbacks

Position yourself either on all fours or on a low bench with one foot on the floor, as illustrated at right. Grasping a dumbbell, start with your arm bent at 90 degrees, then straighten it. By straightening your elbow against load in this position, your triceps are strengthened. Do not raise the weight behind your back. Do as many reps as you can until the muscle action starts to weaken, then do the other side. Keep your back straight.

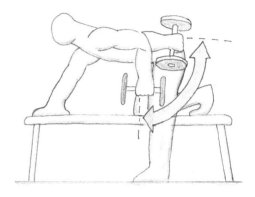

Kickbacks are a good functional fitness aid for using bannisters.

A11 Pushdowns

Pushdowns are a very good **triceps** exercise. It is most important that you do not lean into this exercise – place one foot forward with most of your weight on the back foot and keep your spine straight. Leaning into and over the handgrips is cheating and the exercise will not give you the benefit of isolating the triceps.

The only part of your body that should move with pushdowns is your lower arms from the elbow. For the sake of symmetry, alternate 50/50 between having your left and right foot forward.

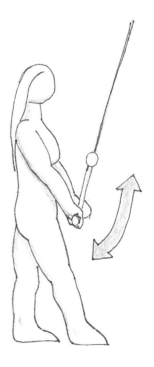

A12   Backward triceps stretch

This is a good **triceps** and **lats** stretch. Place one foot forward and the other back in a wide stance, point your elbow upward, and grasp your wrist behind your head with the other hand. In a smooth and slow motion, pull your upward pointing elbow toward the back of your head without pushing your head forward. You should also feel a good stretch in your calf and hip flexors on the opposite side. Maintain for 20 to 30 seconds, then do the other side.

A variation to this exercise is to hold your elbow (instead of your wrist) and draw it back.

If you have previously dislocated your shoulder, you may not be able to do this, so use with caution and stop if it twinges. You may find **S25 Rotated body stretch** easier to do, which will also stretch your triceps.

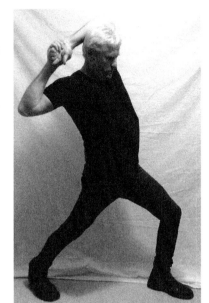

Do not force this stretch. If you have a current lower back injury, avoid doing this exercise.

A13   Biceps curls

Biceps curls directly target the biceps, whether performed with free weights or a lifting machine. They can be done with either an overhand or underhand grip. Usually you will see people favoring the under-hand grip, but try both and see which feels more natural to you.

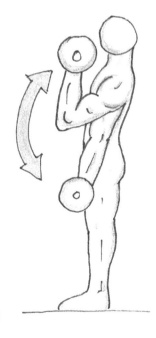

With either grip, keep your spine and your wrists straight. See the diagram at the right for the correct form. It is easier to keep your spine straight if you do biceps curls in the standing position, rather than sitting.

It is important to be aware of the most common mistake that is made when doing biceps curls: hyperextending your lower back to raise the weight (at right). When you are pushing your limits this is a very easy mistake to make. **Always keep your back straight when you lift.**

A14   Thera-Band curls

If you don't have hand weights, you can perform biceps curls using a weights substitute like Thera-Bands. Stand on one end of a Thera-Band and lift your lower arm upward from the elbow as shown.

As with biceps curls with weights, the only part of your body that should move when doing curls with Thera-Bands is your lower arm. Move it straight up and down from the elbow – it should not move sideways.

If you are strong and even the thickest Thera-Band doesn't provide enough resistance, use a double thickness.

Thera-Bands eventually stretch and break but they are cheap and portable – highly useful if you travel for work.

Do not improvise with elasticated luggage straps, as they can injure you if they break.

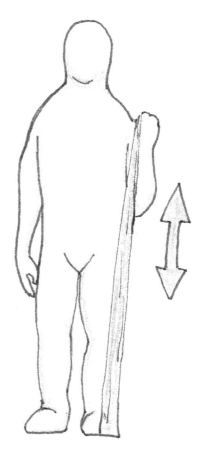

A15   Preacher curls

Preacher curls are the most spine-friendly way of doing biceps curls. Your upper arms are supported as you lift, avoiding any backward leaning that could kink your lower spine. If you find that your preacher curl lifts are less than what you can manage with a standard biceps curl, the difference is how much you were cheating by leaning backward.

If you really want to build your biceps up, preacher curls are the safest and most effective way of doing it.

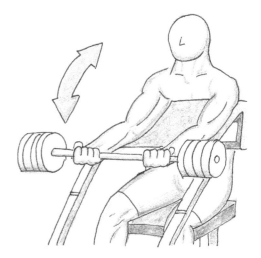

A16   Ball curls

Like preacher curls, ball curls isolate the action of your biceps and keep your back straight too. Press your elbows into the ball to isolate your biceps, and use your elbows as fulcrums to raise and lower the weights.

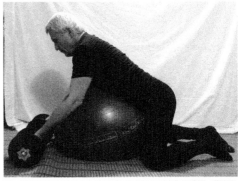

If your knees feel sore in this position, try doing it on a soft rug or low cushion. If you have stiff knees, this exercise may be too difficult for you.

Ensure your Swiss ball is matched to your height and weight and is fully inflated. If you are have not done Ball Curls before, use a lighter weight to start with and be careful not to lift too quickly (so you don't make contact with your head).

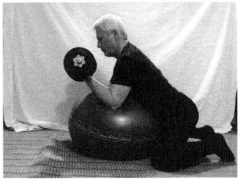

A17   Seated curl

Using smaller hand weights for curls while sitting on a Swiss ball can exercise your biceps and core muscles at the same time. This challenges not only your strength but your balance too. As we get older this matters a lot more; balance exercises are covered more in the Functional Fitness chapter.

Look in a mirror while you do this if it helps. Lifting while you are balanced on a ball is more difficult than you might think.

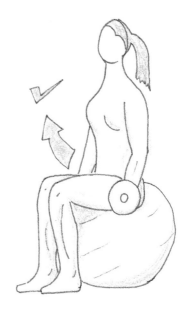

A18   Wrist flex

Support your forearm with the other wrist as shown at right. Without moving any other joints, flex the wrist forward and backward. Much less weight is needed than for curls. Do sets of 6-10 reps.

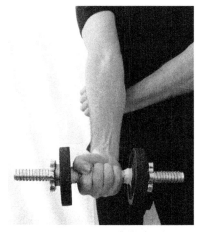

The **wrist flexors** play a helping role in many other exercises, particularly biceps curls, so if you are doing a lot of weight training your wrist flexors are already getting a workout.

Big strong forearms look impressive, but because these are naturally busy muscles, please ensure that you Self Massage and stretch them after doing weights.

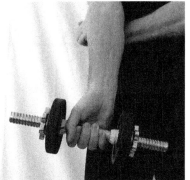

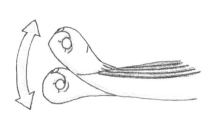

A19   Can flex

Isolating your wrist flexors in a resistance exercise requires lighter weights, which makes it an easy exercise to improvise, in this case with a can of drink over the corner of your work desk. The action is confined to the wrist flexing and straightening with no other movement in the arm. Do 6 to 10 reps.

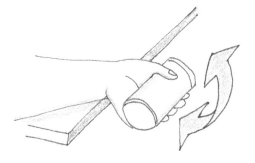

A20 Extensor flex

This exercise is similar to **A18 Wrist flex**, but strengthens the wrist extensors on the opposite side of the forearm.

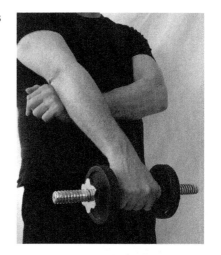

Rest your arm across your other hand and lock your elbow straight, as shown at right. Move your wrist joint backward and then straighten it again. You will need a much lighter weight than for a biceps curl because the wrist extensors are not nearly as strong. Do sets of 6 to 10 reps.

Lower the weight if you have difficulty.

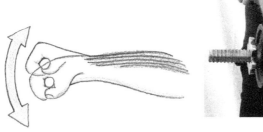

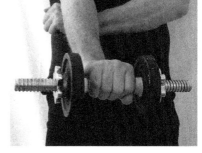

A21 Can extend

This exercise is similar to **A19 Can flex**, but exercises the wrist extensors on the opposite side of the forearm. This time you are palm down. Bend your wrist backward then straighten again. Do 6 to 10 reps off the edge of a desk or bench.

If you are recovering from hand or wrist surgery, a drink can may be all the weight you can handle.

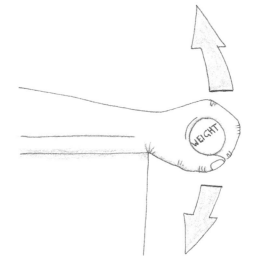

A22   Band flex

You can replace the hand weight in **A18 Wrist flex** with a length of Thera-Band. Stand on one end of the Thera-Band, support your arm (with palm up) with the wrist of the other hand against your chest, and flex your wrist forward. Remember to keep the rest of your arm still: your wrist should be the only part of your body moving in this exercise.

You can also try this exercise doing both sides at once, with one long length of Thera-Band or two shorter ones. Choose a Thera-Band you can do 6 to 10 reps with.

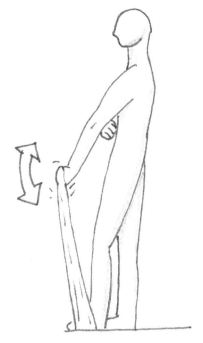

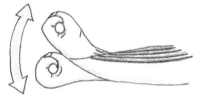

A23   Extensor band flex

While in the same stance as **A22 Band flex**, turn your hand the other way around so your palm is down, and flex your wrist backward to work the extensors.

It is good for the healthy function of the wrist and elbow joints to keep even strength between your wrist extensors and flexors.

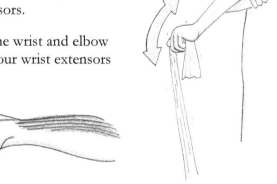

A24   Palm up stretch

Extend one arm straight out in front of you, palm up. Lock the elbow straight and stretch your fingers backward with the other hand. Do this slowly and hold for about 30 seconds, then repeat on the other side.

If this stretch produces any sharp pain, you may have over-stretched or you may be in need of some therapy – try Self Massage techniques **A3** , **A4** and **A5** (pages 96 and 97).

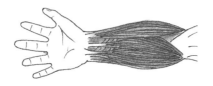

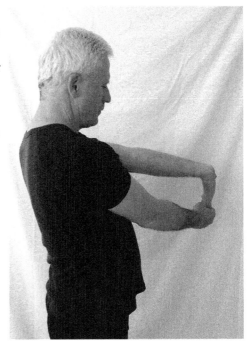

A25   Prayer stretch

Place your palms against each other and push your wrists downward. You should feel your palms, fingers and wrist flexors stretch. Maintain the stretch for at least 20 seconds. This is a good stretch to do after forearm strengthening exercises or working hard with your arms.

Having supple well-stretched hands makes it easier to grasp larger objects. You will find it easier to do this stretch after some Self Massage to your palms.

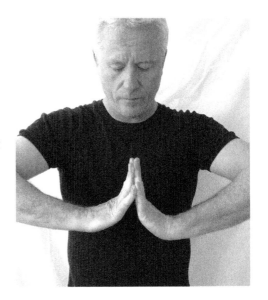

A26   Extensor stretch

Extend your arm with your palm down and your elbow straight. Use the other hand to gently hyper-flex your wrist, as shown at right. Maintain the stretch for 20 to 30 seconds.

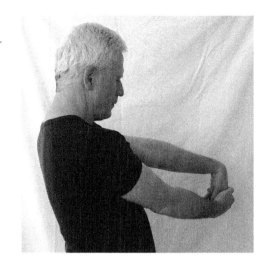

Chronically tight wrist extensors are a common problem for people who work at a computer all day. Players of racquet sports usually have well developed wrist extensors from all the backhanders they hit. If you Self Massage these muscles first with **A6 Ball elbow** and **A7 Elbow ratchet rub** (pages 97 and 98), this stretch will be more productive.

A27   Wrist twist stretch

Turn your palm to face you, and grasp the thumb from behind with the fingers of the other hand. Place the thumb of the grasping hand on the back of the hand being stretched. Gently twist the palm around and downward at the joint. Little pressure is required – just relax into the stretch and wait 20 to 30 seconds.

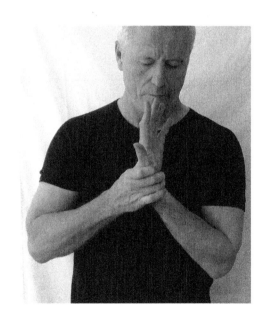

As with any stretch, don't use sudden movements, rocking or jerking. You will feel the stretch when you get the right angle and relax into it.

This stretch is used extensively in jiu jitsu and aikido training. It is easy to do sitting at your desk or waiting for traffic lights to change.

A28   Backward finger stretch

Each of your fingers has its own muscles attached to it. In this exercise, simply stretch back each finger individually.

If you want your fingers to stay nimble, you have to stretch them. The muscles that bend and straighten fingers are in the forearms, attached to the fingers via tendons.

The tendons and the fascia under the skin of the palms will also feel more relaxed and supple from this exercise.

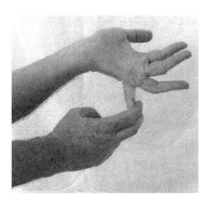

A29   Backward thumb stretch

Cross your wrists over as shown and stretch your thumb sideways and backward away from the palm. You will feel your thumb and lower palm stretch when you are in the correct position.

This is a nice easy, controlled way to stretch the muscles and fascia of the thumb. If you are picking heavy objects up all day like a bricklayer would, this can relieve tension in your hands. This should feel good – if it hurts, you are pushing too hard.

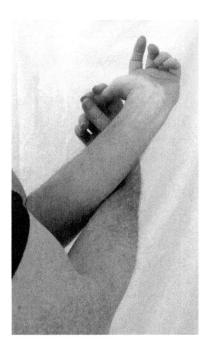

A30   Silly putty flex

If you need to strengthen your grip, Theraputty is a useful exercise tool to achieve this with. Unlike the old-fashioned wood and steel hand squeezers, Theraputty is a Plasticine-like substance especially designed for hand physiotherapy. Unlike Plasticine, Theraputty does not feel greasy, will not stain your clothes and will bounce like a rubber ball if you roll it up.

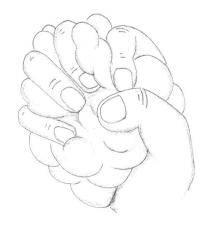

Theraputty is fun to play with and very tactile. Squeeze it, work it side to side in your hand and squelch it between your fingers. By working the Theraputty in every possible direction, you will be able to exercise the fine intrinsic muscles in your hand.

A31   Finger spread flex

This is as low-tech as it gets. Stretch a rubber band around the end phalanges of your fingers and then splay them apart. After about 10 to 20 reps, the muscles on the upper side of your forearms should feel like they have been exercised.

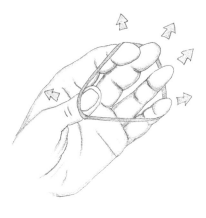

Do this slowly so the rubber band doesn't roll down your fingers.

A32   Thumb to fingers

This exercise is for hand dexterity. No force is required, only the touching together of the thumb to each of the fingertips. Hand surgeons often instruct their patients to do this exercise to assist in post-surgical rehabilitation.

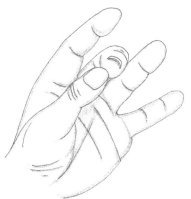

You will find further information about the care of your hands in the Reflexology chapter.

12.4 RISK ARM & HAND EXERCISES

Dips are a popular triceps strengthening exercise that you may have seen many times, but they are hard on your shoulders and place your spine in a bent position. Push-ups and kickbacks will strengthen your triceps much more safely.

The similar look of this exercise to gymnasts using parallel bars has no doubt helped lead to its popularity (using parallel bars isn't very good for your shoulders either).

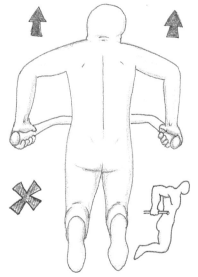

The **Shoulder Press** and **Incline Press** can injure your shoulders, lower back and neck.

Weight lifting is a good example of a sport that can really take a toll on your body, as it compresses joints from your wrists to your ankles. Use of weights can be very effective strengthening exercise, but not when used like this.

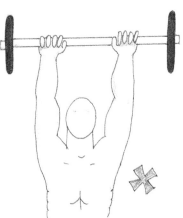

Sometimes you will see people in the gym doing curls as shown at right, even in body building magazines. Bending your back with your hips in a rotated position while turning your head might create an interesting photograph, but it is not a good way to do biceps curls.

Lift with a straight back always.

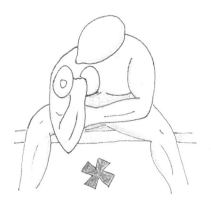

13 LOWER BODY

The muscles of the lower body are amongst your biggest and strongest. They are also the most influential in your posture and balance. Your core muscles are found mostly in this part of your anatomy.

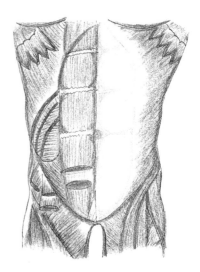

The core muscles hold our spines straight. The primary core muscles are found in the front of the body, in the pelvic floor, in the back, and deep inside the abdominal cavity. At the time of writing this book, core strength is very topical because it has become widely understood only fairly recently.

This chapter describes exercises that promote core strength – exercises like planking, where muscles are flexed in a stationary position and held still for a short period of time. Goodman's Foundation Training exercises in Chapter 7 should also be referred to.

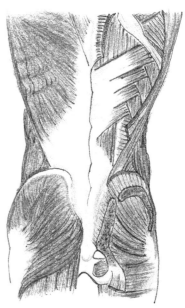

Muscular tension in the lower body is a major cause of back pain, not only from tight back muscles but also from the muscles in your hips and buttocks. Try the Self Massage techniques in this chapter to help with these problems. There are additional techniques in the Advanced Self Massage and Self Acupressure & Shiatsu chapters that you can try after you have mastered the easier ones.

Back pain is more common during cold weather, so keeping your lower back warm and covered will assist your Self Massage efforts. As with Self Massage to other parts of your body, these techniques should feel good, so don't wait until you are in pain to do them. Do them with your exercises in the morning each day.

If you are suffering from an acute lower back injury, go lightly and desist if your pain worsens.

13.1 PRIMARY CORE MUSCLES OF THE LOWER BODY

The primary core muscles consist of four groups. The **multifidus** is located along the entire length of the spine. It is like an overlapping chain of small individual muscles that help join and support the individual vertebrae (backbones). It runs from your sacrum to the top of your neck. The multifidus of the lower back is illustrated at right.

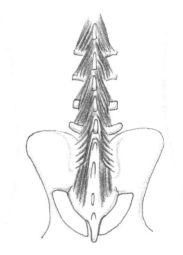

No other muscle group articulates so closely with the spinal column, so it is easy to see why it is of primary importance to our posture and core strength.

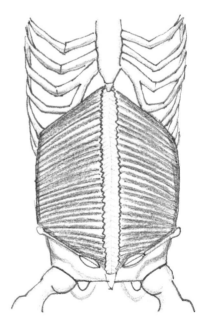

The **transverse abdominis** is illustrated at right. It sucks your belly in sideways and frontward when it is flexed. It is the deepest of the four layers of abdominal muscle and provides a more complete muscular covering over your abdomen than the other more superficial layers (internal and external obliques and rectus abdominis, discussed below).

The transverse abdominis forms a muscular wall that wraps around your mid-section. To engage it, you need to suck your belly in as you tense. Unlike the six-pack (rectus abdominis), it is not visible when flexed.

The **pelvic floor** supports our internal organs from underneath. It is like a sling with sphincters in it that close like a drawstring bag. At right is the top view of the pelvic floor muscles.

Women tend to suffer at younger ages than men from weaknesses here because of bearing children.

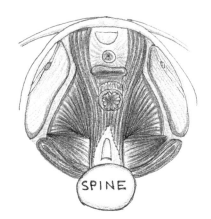

Perhaps the most intriguing feature of your core is its lid, the **diaphragm**. The diaphragm is dome shaped and has four apertures in it. Your esophagus (food pipe), one of the largest veins (inferior vena cava), largest artery (aorta) and spine pass through these apertures. The diaphragm is your main breathing muscle – it is impossible to breathe without it.

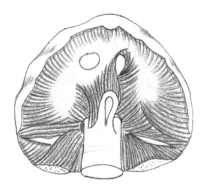

The multifidus vertically supports your core, the pelvic floor supports it from beneath and the transverse abdominis is the wall around your core. When the diaphragm contracts, it creates a downward pressure onto your abdomen.

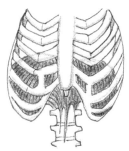

As a result, when all four of these muscle groups are strong and work together, they create a firm support for your body's structure, like a muscular pressurized piston and cylinder. Together, the primary core muscles support your lower back in all directions. Planking (page 118) and the Goodman's exercises in Chapter 7 emphasize the synchronous use of these muscles.

13.2 SECONDARY MUSCLES OF THE LOWER BODY

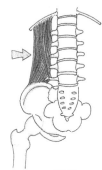

The **quadratus lumborum** (or "QL") helps the body bend sideways when flexed on one side. When flexed, they protect the spine from a side-on impact.

The QLs become sore from poor posture. If you find twisting from your waist difficult, these muscles are probably stiff and need loosening.

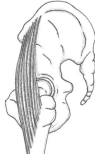

The **tensor fasciae latae** (TFL) is one of the muscles of the **hip flexor** group, located on the front of your hips. When contracted they help other hip flexor muscles tip your body forward at the hips.

Your hip flexors tend to shorten if not frequently stretched, a common problem with sit-down jobs. Shortened hip flexors cause lower back and hip pain.

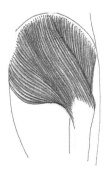

The **gluteal** muscles, or butt muscles, are the biggest muscles in the body. They help your hamstrings move your thigh backward and deliver most of the power you need for walking and running up steep hills. Your gluteals also thrust your hips forward. The gluteals engage when you arch backward and when you stand up. When they weaken, it is harder to stand up.

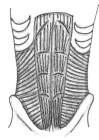

The **rectus abdominis**, commonly known as your "six-pack," forms part of the outer layer of abdominal muscle. The **obliques** are to the side of the rectus abdominis, with the external obliques on the top and the internal obliques underneath and oriented at right angles to them.

Your six-pack and internal and external obliques work quite cooperatively. The six-pack bends you forward and the obliques enable you to twist and bend sideways. Belly dancers control these muscles well.

13.3 SELF MASSAGE OF THE LOWER BODY

B1   Lumbar rub

If you have ever done tai chi, you may recognize this as a warm-up exercise. Stand with your feet a shoulder's width apart and rub your lower back vigorously. Sometimes a bit of warmth can give a lot of relief. You can also rub with the backs of your hands if it is easier for you.

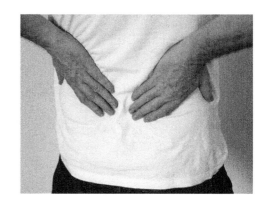

B2   Lumbar knuckles

Stand with your feet a shoulder's width apart and use your knuckles to deliver deeper pressure into those stiff lower body muscles. If you extend your bent index finger joint, you can apply more focused pressure in those extra-stiff spots. Apply pressure from beside the muscle and from behind too.

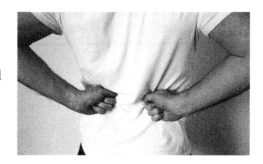

B3   Seated lumbar knuckles

You can apply firmer pressure than **B2 Lumbar knuckles** if you use a wall or a chair. (Make sure that the chair you use has a strong back.) With your arms behind you, use your body weight (instead of your arm muscles) to apply pressure against your knuckles, using the wall or chair back to push against. You can either move your knuckles around (with your wrists against the chair back) or use static pressure over a relieving pressure point. Use the illustration at right as a guide to the area that you can Self Massage.

This is a good Self Massage technique to do while sitting down at work.

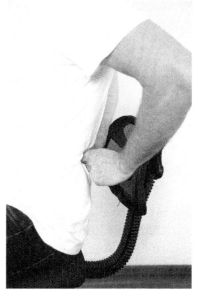

115

B4 Lumbar wall lean

Stand side-on to a wall with one foot forward and one back. Bend your elbow out to the side and brace it against the wall. Apply pressure with your extended knuckle by gradually leaning sideways into the wall. **Do not do this abruptly**. Hold the pressure for 15 to 30 seconds while relaxing your lower back into the pressure. Then do the other side.

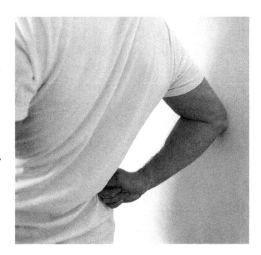

You should only try this technique if you found **B2 Lumbar knuckles** and **B3 Seated lumbar knuckles** comfortable to do. This technique can be used to apply greater pressure to the muscles of your lower back.

B5 Wall ball hip

Place your feet about a shoulder's width apart, positioned diagonally next to a wall. Position a ball between your hip and the wall, so that the ball can roll along the fleshy part of the side of your hip. Lean sideways into the wall and relax into the pressure, taking most of your weight on the foot furthest from the wall. You can steady yourself with a hand on the wall if you need to. Turn your hips back and forth to help loosen these muscles.

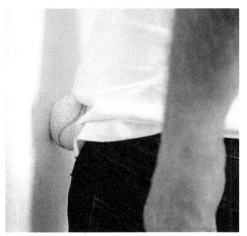

The muscles toward the front of your hips are prone to shortening from sitting for long periods. Try sitting cross-legged on the floor – if you can't, it is time to take better care of these muscles.

You can further relieve tension in these front hip muscles by stretching them after Self Massaging using exercises like **B21 Standing groin stretch** and **B22 Kneeling groin stretch** (page 124). Sometimes, loosening these muscles even if they are not sore can bring relief to lower back pain.

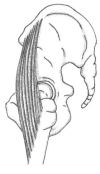

B6   Upper thigh rub

While sitting, use a hand-held massage tool or your fist to rub the muscles on the top of the thigh. If you have never been massaged here before, you may be surprised how stiff and sensitive it can feel.

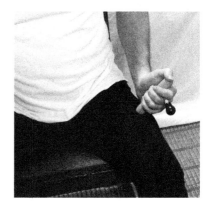

If you find lifting one or both legs difficult while walking up stairs, your hip flexors may be the cause. The more often you do this, the more your hips should free up. The muscle tissue is quite deep here so use firm pressure if it is comfortable to do so.

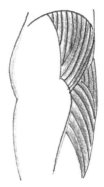

Your upper thigh and anterior (front) hip muscles should be relaxed while sitting in this position. If you find that the muscle is not sensitive but not soft either, it may be because it is a bit numb, as sometimes happens with chronically stiff muscles.

Probe around and spend a few minutes on each side, concentrating on the most unyielding areas. Gradually the muscles will start to loosen and you will feel a pleasant looseness afterward. Be patient for results, as these are thick, strong muscles. Persistence pays off.

Self Massage of the lower body helps make lower body exercises easier to do.

13.4 Core strength exercises

B7   Planking

Lie face down with your hands under your shoulders. Keep your legs and back straight, raise yourself into a pushup position, and hold this position for 30 seconds if you can. The most important thing with planking is to keep your body as straight and steady as possible. Stop when you start to weaken. As your core strengthens, you will last longer. This is a good isometric exercise for your abs, legs and back.

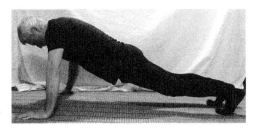

If you cannot raise your body in a straight line, plank on your knees instead of your toes, using the starting position for **S12 Knee push-up** (page 80).

B8   Elbow planking

If you find **B7 Planking** easy, this variation on your elbows is more strenuous and exercises your abs more deeply. Keep your eyes looking straight down, elbows beneath shoulders, core engaged and pressing your breath down into your abdomen. Keep your body as straight as you can and maintain the position for as long as you can remain steady.

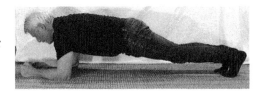

You may find this exercise easier if you use some padding under your elbows.

B9   Supine pedaling

Lie flat on your back and pedal an imaginary exercise bike, with your legs at roughly a 45-degree angle from the floor. This exercise works your obliques as well as your six-pack because the pedaling motion rocks your body from side to side. Spread your arms to the side to steady yourself – this will help you do the exercise properly.

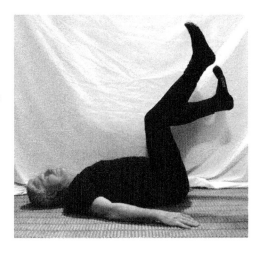

B10 Bird dog stretch/strength

The bird dog strengthens your back as it stretches your front. It is not only a core and stretching exercise but is also good for your balance. Starting on all fours, extend and stretch one arm forward and the opposite leg backward. Maintain this posture for as long as you can while maintaining the correct posture with a straight spine. Then do the other side. Do this on a yoga mat or soft rug for comfort. (The lower illustration is your starting position, the upper figure is the actual exercise.)

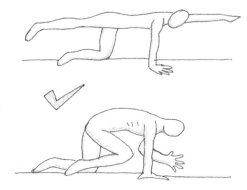

B11 Side planking

This exercise works your core with an emphasis on the obliques at the side of your abdomen. (The strength of the side muscles is as important as that of the front and back.) You must have a straight back to do this, with your shoulders and hips in a straight line too. Maintain the position until you tire, then do the other side. To increase the difficulty, do this with your arm straight and your weight on your palm.

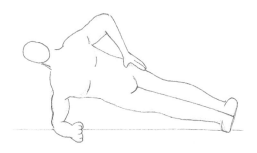

B12 Side knee planks

If **B11 Side planking** is too difficult, try this easier variation: place your weight on your knees instead of keeping your legs outstretched. The same muscles are used but with less intensity. It is important to keep your back dead straight. Do both sides.

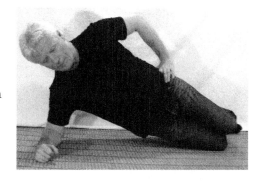

If you find getting onto the floor to do plank exercises difficult, go to the Goodman's exercises in Chapter 7 (pages 47 to 50). The Goodman's exercises are done standing up and are just as useful for core strength.

B13 Rolling ball planks

Rolling ball planks are a good alternative to crunches. This exercise works your six-pack (rectus abdominis) and your lats. Keep your back straight while you roll your forearms against the Swiss ball, tipping your body forward from your hips until it is parallel to the floor. Hold this position until you start to lose form. **A few slow reps are more effective than numerous faster ones.**

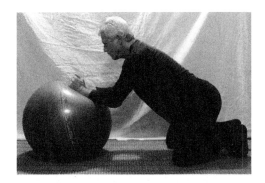

Cushion your knees for comfort and ensure that the ball has some grip on the floor.

This exercise will help with your balance and proprioception as well as exercising your abs and shoulders.

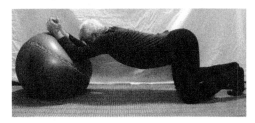

B14 Sitting straight

Simply sitting on a Swiss ball will exercise your core muscles. This is a great core exercise and improves your sitting posture. Because the ball is round, you can only sit still and feel balanced if you are perfectly straight. As you get used to sitting on the ball this way, you will start to sit more upright on ordinary chairs too.

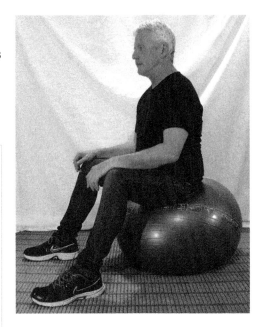

Several years ago I worked with a lady who had very slouchy posture and frequently complained of back pain. This person did not like exercising, so it surprised me when a colleague managed to talk L into taking a Swiss ball home to use as her new lounge chair. A month or so later, L's sitting posture had improved enormously and she was not getting any lower back pain. All this from sitting on her ball each day after work, watching the TV before bed.

B15 The cat & camel stretch

These are two different yoga asanas but they work well when used together. Start on your hands and knees, with your back straight. Adopt the camel asana, with your chin tucked in and mid back stretched as high as you can, and hold for 10 seconds. Then adopt cat asana by arching backward, pushing your belly forward and chin stretched forward, and hold for 10 seconds. This is usually safe for touchy backs but if it hurts, stop doing it and get medical advice. Stop when you start to tire.

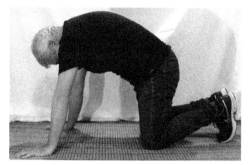

If your knees get sore, you can use a firm bed.

These asanas are amongst the safer and less demanding stretches if you have back pain. Like all exercises though, if you feel awkward or in pain doing this, stop immediately.

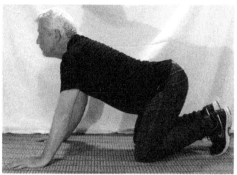

B16 Bridging

This exercise strengthens your lower back. Lie on your back with your knees bent and your feet flat on the floor. From that position, raise your hips upward so as to form a straight line from your knees to your shoulders. Your weight is on your feet and upper back. Do not hyperextend by pushing your belly up too far. (Look sideways in a mirror to see if you are straight.) Maintain this position for about 20 seconds. If your back or neck hurts, stop.

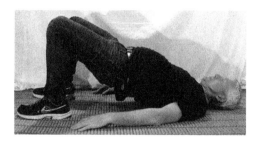

13.5 LOWER BODY STRETCHES

B17 Supine knee rocking

Lie on your back on the floor or on a firm bed, with your arms straight out and parallel with your shoulders. Bend your knees up with ankles together as shown and start slowly rocking your hips side to side by moving your knees together.

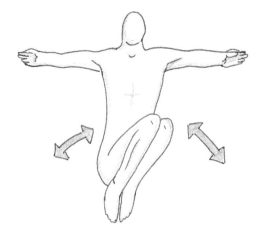

This is one of the safer, less demanding stretches for your lower back. If your back is too sensitive to do this you should seek professional assistance from your doctor or bodyworker.

B18 Flexor & butt stretch

This is a dual-purpose exercise. Lie on a sturdy table and let one leg hang limply off the edge to stretch the hip flexors. Draw the other knee up to the chest to stretch your butt muscles (gluteals). If you have a high enough bed, you can do this off its end. Hold for 20 to 30 seconds and then do the other side. Stop this if it hurts.

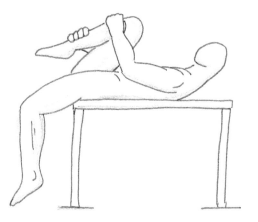

B19 Pigeon stretch

This yoga asana stretches the abductors on the outside of the thigh, in addition to the butt muscles (gluteals). Support your upper bodyweight on your hands, with arms straight and with your body bent upright from your hips. One leg is straight out behind, the other is bent at the knee pointing forward and tucked beneath you. It is most important that you can feel the floor on the **side** of your forward bent leg and that the front of the trailing leg is against the floor.

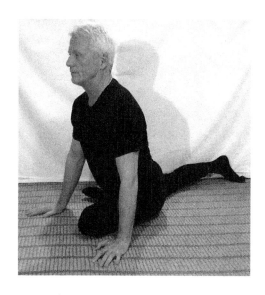

If your butt muscles are too stiff for this, Self Massage them and use a less demanding butt stretch like **B18 Flexor and butt stretch**.

B20 Standing butt stretch

Bend one leg and rest its outer side on a sturdy bench or desk, ensuring that it is at the right height. You may need a lower table if you are a little on the short side or your hip is quite stiff. (Never attempt this on anything with wheels or with loose objects like books on top of it.)

Balance with your body weight supported on one foot and your hands. You should feel a stretch from your butt muscles (gluteals) along the outside of your thigh to your knee. You can lean forward to increase the stretch. If you are already fairly flexible, this is a convenient stretch you can do at work.

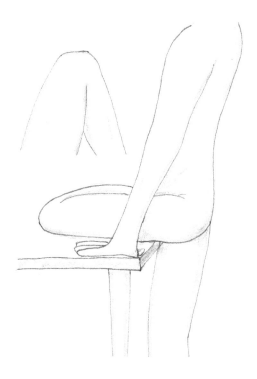

This is not the easiest butt stretch to do, so don't continue if you can't balance and relax into the stretch.

B21 Standing groin stretch

Stand facing a wall, with one foot almost touching the wall and the other stretched backward behind you. Extend your arms forward and place your palms against the wall. By bending your leading leg forward, your height drops and your back leg stretches at the groin and calf.

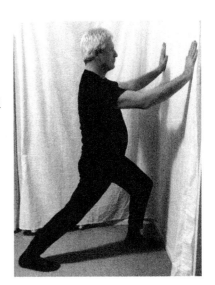

Keep your arms almost straight and **do not** lean forward, but keep your body upright or even leaning slightly backward, in order to ensure that the hip flexors are stretched. Maintain the stretch for at least 20 seconds, then do the other side. If you position your body correctly, this exercise should stretch your groin and/or calf muscles.

Keep your shoulders vertically aligned with or slightly behind your hips. If you lean forward, the stretch won't work.

B22 Kneeling groin stretch

Place one foot forward with knee bent and the other leg back behind you with its knee on the floor (use a thin cushion for comfort). Keep your body upright as you push your hips forward with your hands. Your leading knee bends more as you do this. Your relaxed back leg should feel that it is stretching in the groin and upper thigh area. For balance, it is fine to use a hand to steady yourself on the wall or a solid piece of furniture. Maintain the stretch for 30 seconds and then do the other side.

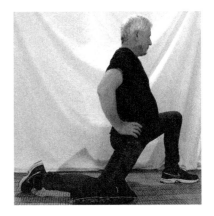

Tight groin muscles can produce lower back pain. In an increasingly sedentary workforce, these are important stretches to do.

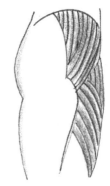

Like **B21 Standing groin stretch**, this is a leg as well as a groin stretch. It looks very similar to a lunge, as your body is placed in a similar position. Lunges, however, emphasize strengthening the thigh, not stretching the groin.

B23 Knee to ankle butt stretch

Lie on your back on the floor or a firm bed. Bend one knee up and place your foot flat on the floor, then lift your other leg to rest its ankle on the outside of your upward pointing knee. Reach down to place both hands around the shin (as shown in the illustration) and pull your upper body toward your lower leg. You should feel a stretch in your butt muscle (gluteals) as you do this.

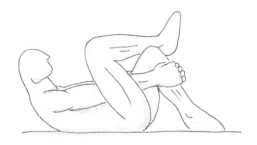

Hold the stretch for 20 seconds and then do the other side. If it hurts your back or leg, cease immediately.

B24 Ball bird dog stretch/strength

This is a variation on **B10 Bird dog stretch** that is easier on the knees and has a higher neuromotor benefit. Position yourself on your belly on a Swiss ball so that you are balancing most of your body weight on it, and stretch out one arm and the opposite leg. You should have relatively little weight on the hand and foot that are on the floor. Use a Swiss ball that is suitable for your size and weight. Alternate both sides and stop when you start to tire.

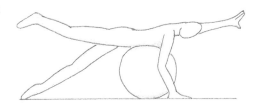

B25 Bowed side stretch

Cross your feet over (as shown at right) and hold a post or doorway with one arm. Reach as high as you can with the other arm to touch the wall directly above your head, stretching the lateral (side) muscles of the shoulder, upper arm, mid-back, hip and thigh.

Keep your hips and head straight, not turned to the side. Let your relaxed hip lead the stretch.

All the stretching should be felt on your side. If you cannot feel the stretch along the shaded area of the illustration, it is probably because you are not reaching for the wall directly above your head. Keep your shoulders and hips at right angles to the wall as you lean sideways.

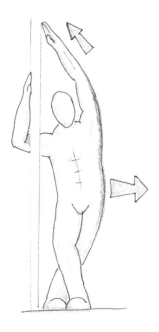

13.6 RISKY LOWER BODY EXERCISES

Sit-ups and **crunches** will strengthen your six-pack but they can also cause and worsen back and hip pain. Planking and Goodman's Foundation Training will not only do a better job at strengthening your abs, but will strengthen your lower back and thighs too – without the back pain.

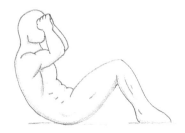

The **Resisted Back Arch** can bend you backward too far, especially if your reps are done rapidly. If you already suffer from lower back pain this can make it worse. It is like a reverse crunch and, like the crunch, is no good for your spinal discs. Bridging (page 121) with a straight back is a safer and more effective exercise to strengthen your butt and lower back.

When lifting anything, even if it's your own body weight, always do so with a straight spine.

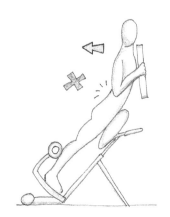

Hip machines, though popular in women's gyms, can give you lower back pain and stiffness. Despite the fact that many fitness trainers do not approve of hip machines, they still seem to keep popping up around the place. Unfortunately, you cannot make the assumption that you should use the equipment just because it is there.

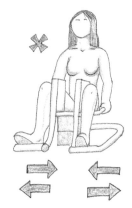

The **cobra** is a yoga asana that is usually fairly easy to do when young. As we age, the lowest part of the spine starts to get disc narrowing and hyperextending becomes much more difficult. There are safer and better ways to stretch your lower body and thighs.

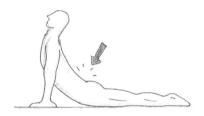

14 LEGS & FEET

We use the muscles in our legs and feet a great deal, usually in activities that require little conscious thought like walking, climbing stairs, standing and getting on and off chairs.

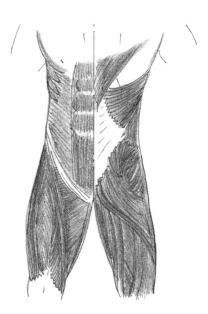

Muscular tension gradually builds up in these muscle groups until our legs and feet start to stiffen, cause pain and slow us down. Usually stiffness and pain will affect one side first. When this happens, it causes us to walk and stand unevenly, which then affects the lower back and hips. As we continue to favor one side, we overuse the other leg, which then develops new problems because we are walking too heavily on the "good side." The problem spreads and intensifies.

Most of the muscle and joint pain problems I have encountered with my clients' legs and feet over the years have not been from accidental trauma. They have developed gradually from being overweight, neglecting to exercise (stretching in particular) and poor posture.

Cartilage wear in the knees and hips is inevitable with aging, but the degree to which it affects the quality of our lives is very much affected by exercise, getting massage, posture and diet – things we do have some control over.

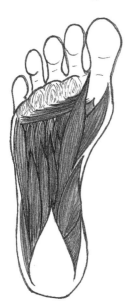

Pain and weakness in our legs and feet is usually followed by weight gain, which then makes everything worse. There is no part of the body that needs Self Massage more than our hips, legs and feet. Most cardio involves the use of our legs and feet. If stiff legs make cardio too painful, regularly Self Massaging your legs could be the key to getting fitter faster and without injury.

Think of your feet as the structural foundation of your body and your legs as the piers that hold it up. A strong and stable building can't be supported well by weak and uneven foundations.

Your legs and feet can be highly susceptible to repetitive strain injuries from things like running, lifting, sport and poor posture. It really can take you by surprise when a simple movement or task that you have performed hundreds of times without mishap suddenly and painfully gives way one day.

You might have a sharp deep pain in your knee that is totally unrelated to trauma or joint disease, caused by an adjacent stiff muscle that does not feel that uncomfortable at all. There have been numerous times I have seen clients with knee pain that their doctor could find no cause of using scans or even arthroscopic surgery. The problem was actually muscular.

For example, the vastus medialis (above the inner knee, and one of the four quadriceps muscles) will sometimes be related to such knee pain. When massaged or Self Massaged, you may notice an improvement in how your knee feels. Tight calves can likewise cause heel pain, and tight thigh muscles can cause your hip and lower back to hurt. It may surprise you to know that you have relatively few nerve endings in your legs. This is why the exact source of your pain can be hard to locate.

Most forms of cardiovascular exercise emphasize the use of your legs and feet. Strengthening and stretching your legs and feet is important for your posture and for the health of your ankles, knees and hips.

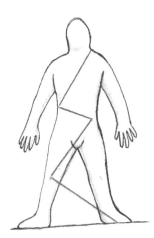

Your posture can become very crooked if you favor one side over the other because of foot or leg pain. Good osteopaths, physiotherapists, chiropractors and massage therapists recognize this relationship, which usually manifests as a diagonal compensation that can affect you along the full length of your body.

Symmetrical muscle tone and flexibility in your feet, legs and hips will improve your posture. Exercising your legs and feet regularly with stretching, strengthening, neuromotor and cardiovascular exercise will give you more to look forward to as you age. Don't let them seize up.

If exercise or massage worsens calf pain, see your doctor, as you may have a DVT.

14.1 MUSCLES OF THE LEGS AND FEET

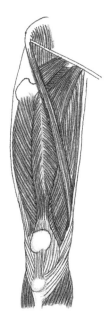

The **quadriceps** ("quads") above the knee and the **hip flexors** at the top of the thigh straighten your knee and raise your leg frontward from your hip (diagram at left). When you walk, run, climb stairs, and kick a ball, these muscles are in action. Doing these things becomes difficult when these muscles are weak, stiff or injured.

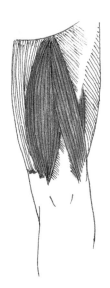

The **hamstrings** on the back of your upper leg (at right) and the **gluteals** (butt muscles) above them work together to raise your leg backward from your hip and to bend your knee. The hamstrings commonly tear in runners because of sudden hyperextension of the leg.

The quads and hamstrings have opposing agonist/antagonist actions.

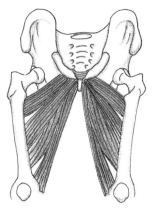

The **hip adductors** (at left) are the muscles on your inner thigh that move your legs together. They help us move sideways and keep us upright. We use them when we kick with the inner edge of the foot. They are stiff on most people because they never bother to stretch them. Some of the deeper muscles of the inner thigh connect directly to the spine, and Self Massage of these muscles can help ease back and knee pain.

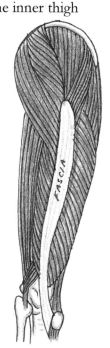

Your hip adductors are quite bulky and are definitely used by some more than others – soccer players and martial artists, for instance, create much power in their kicks using the adductors. When these muscles become tight, it can affect your balance by narrowing your walking and standing gait.

The **hip abductors** on your outer thigh (at right) move your legs apart. They help us move sideways and to kick with the outer edge of the foot.

Together your abductors and adductors form an agonist/antagonist pairing. Many elderly people experience the fear of falling because their balance is not good – having good adductors and abductors steadies sideways movement and improves balance.

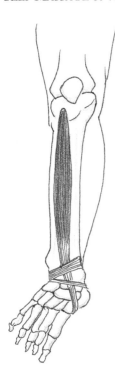

The **tibialis anterior** and **tibialis posterior** ("tibs") point your toes up (at left). We use them when we walk, run, kick, climb stairs and put our shoes and socks on. These muscles get tight when we walk fast.

Right next to your tibs along the outer side of your lower leg are your **peroneus** muscles (at right). The boney bump on the outside of your knee is the upper attachment point for the peroneus, which runs down to your ankle. The peroneus is a very difficult muscle to stretch so the only way it can be loosened is with massage. The peroneus moves our ankles outward and stabilizes their position. If you have a tendency to roll over on your ankles, Self Massage them with **L12 Peroneus roll** (page 135).

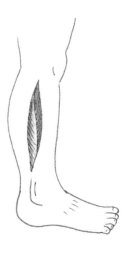

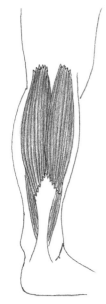

The **gastrocnemius** and **soleus** (calf muscles) point your toes down. They are activated when we walk, run, jump, climb stairs and stand on our toes. The calves commonly tear on runners when suddenly breaking into a sprint. Your calves act as shock absorbers when you step and jump down.

Together the tibs and the calves form an agonist/antagonist relationship.

Last but not least, your humble foot probably works harder than any other body part. Essential for walking and running, the muscles in the sole of the foot perform an important role with balance. Bad shoes wreck feet, but fortunately feet respond very well to regular massage.

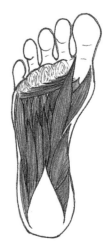

14.2 SELF MASSAGE OF THE LEGS AND FEET

L1 Sole roll

This is one of the most well known ways to Self Massage. Use a small ball (such as a golf ball) and roll it under your sole. **Do this sitting up not standing**. If you are on your feet a lot, this is something you should do every day. This technique can also bring relief to plantar fasciitis, a painful condition of the sole of the foot. If your feet are sore or inflamed, roll a bumpy or ridged frozen water bottle beneath them instead of a ball.

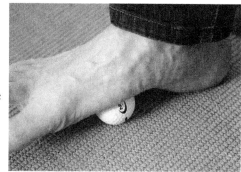

L2 Sole pluck

This technique is like the opposite of **L1 Sole roll**. Instead of pressing, gently pinch and lift your sole and toes in a light plucking manner. This allows your blood to circulate more efficiently and it should feel relieving. If it is painful you are pinching too hard. Apply **L1** to the soft skin on your sole and this exercise to the tougher skin that you walk on.

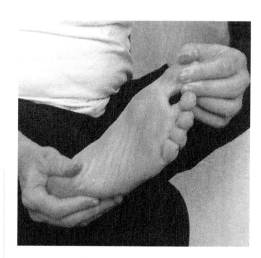

> Sitting or lying with your feet elevated above the height of your knees can relieve sore feet too, by allowing pooled blood to drain back into your legs. As we get older, our circulation is less efficient and needs help like this.

L3 Knee and calf rub

Lie on your back and bend one knee up. Rest the calf of your other leg on the point of your knee and move it back and forth. Self Massaging the lower part of your calf can relieve foot pain, while Self Massaging the upper part can relieve knee discomfort. You can do this in bed or on the floor. If this hurts your knee, stop.

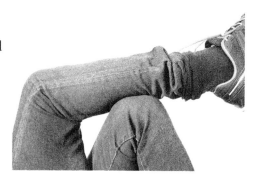

You can also do this while sitting up. Hold your massaged leg with your hands for extra stability if you like. **Do not apply over varicose veins**.

L4   Fist to outer calf

Sit upright and bend your knee so your foot is resting on the floor beside you and you can reach straight down to your calf. Lock your arm straight and lean from your shoulder downward to apply vertical pressure on your calf muscles with your fist or hand-held massage tool. Do both sides.

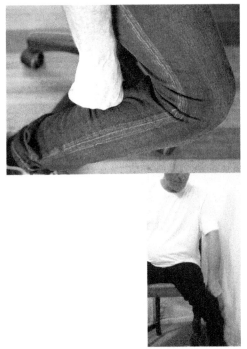

It is best to work from the bottom up to give venous return (darker blood going back to your heart) maximum assistance. Exercising your calves assists venous return too. Regular calf Self Massage can assist calf flexibility.

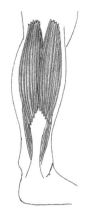

Right fist to right calf, left fist to left calf.

L5   Fist to inner calf

Sit upright and move your foot sideways so your lower leg is angled in front of you. With one hand supporting your balance on your leg or chair, reach down to massage your inner calf muscle with your opposite fist or hand-held massage tool. You can brace your elbow against the inside of your other leg for better leverage. **Keep your back as straight as possible.** Your head should be above the heel of your massaged leg.

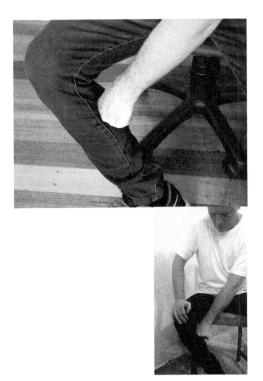

Right fist to left calf, left fist to right calf.

> **Do not apply L4 or L5 directly over varicose veins.**

132

L6 Knuckle to calf

Sit upright, raise your foot, and rest it sideways on the other knee. Using an extended knuckle or massage tool, press along the inner calf muscle from your ankle toward your knee. Use your other hand to hold your ankle to steady your leg.

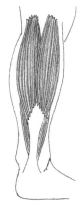

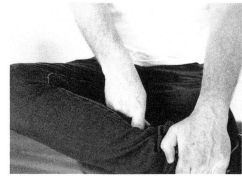

Work close to the bone but not on it. **Do not apply over varicose veins.**

L7 Elbow to thigh

Sit upright with your legs apart. Use the point of your elbow to palpate the muscle in the middle of the front of your thigh (rectus femoris, one of the four quadriceps muscles). Work from the knee up to the hip. If you are a runner or cyclist this can be very helpful to do. For best results, empty your pockets first.

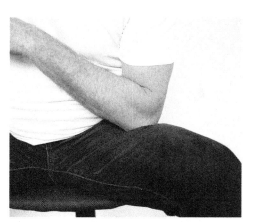

Rest your other hand on your other leg for balance.

This muscle's natural action is to raise your leg in front of you. If you have trouble raising one or both of your legs to put your pants or socks on of a morning, stiffness in this muscle or the hip flexors above it may be the cause.

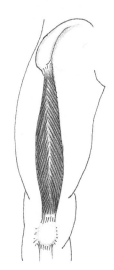

Self Massaging this muscle can help you climb stairs or ladders more easily. It can also help free up stiff knees.

L8   Adductor press

Sit upright with your legs apart. Lean forward and angle your forearm between the open thighs. Brace your fist on the opposite leg and use your elbow to Self Massage the lower end of the hip adductors just above the inner side of the knee. Work along the whole length of the muscle.

For a more advanced adductor technique, see **X15 Lateral thigh roll** (page 160).

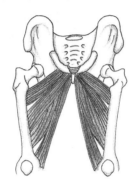

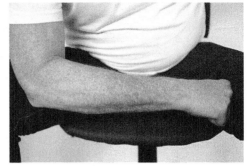

L9   Upper thigh rub

While sitting, use a hand-held massage tool or your fist to rub the muscles on the top of the thigh. This is essentially the same technique as **B6 Upper thigh rub** except that you go lower down your quadriceps. Apply firm downward pressure with your fist or massage tool to create a "good pain" sensation.

You won't need much force to find quite tender spots. Firmer quad techniques can be found in the Advanced Self Massage chapter.

If you want to do this to bare skin, use massage oil or skin moisturizer.

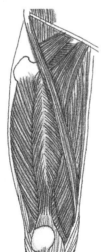

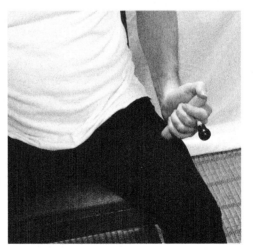

L10 Ball thigh press

Sit on a chair and place a ball under the middle of the back of your thigh, in the groove between the inner and outer sides of the hamstring muscle. Move the ball along the groove of the hamstrings and straighten the leg from the knee a few times in each position. This will loosen your hamstrings as well as give your quads some resistance exercise.

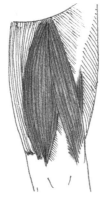 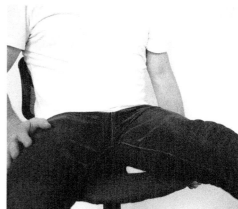

L11 Hamstring ball

Sit on a firm seat and place a ball under your thigh. Lean forward and backward to apply pressure to the hamstring, changing the position of the ball to cover as much area as possible. Moving the ball even slightly backward, forward or sideways can make a difference to how this works and feels. If any particular position feels good, rest there for longer.

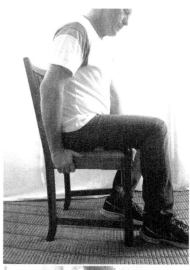

L12 Peroneus roll

Sit on the floor or your bed, bend one knee up and turn the knee inward. Roll a walking stick with a cardboard tube around it up the side of your lower leg. The tube helps it roll more easily without chafing your leg. Tubes of similar length and width like PVC conduit can also be used. Place a cushion behind your back for comfort.

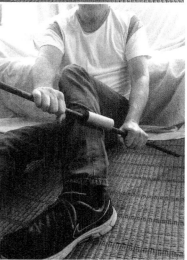

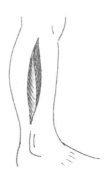

L13 Ant tib roll

Place your hands on the back of a strong stable chair for balance. Place a ball between the seat and the anterior tibialis muscle. Slowly roll the ball back and forth along the muscle. This may feel a bit intense if you have not done it before so go lightly at first. Use greater pressure when rolling the ball upward toward the knee than on the return down stroke.

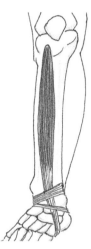

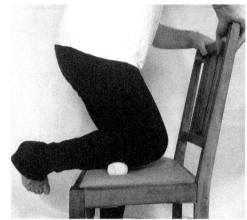

L14 Tibial roll

Sit on the floor or your bed and bend one knee up in front of you. Use a walking stick with a cardboard tube around it to roll up the front of your lower leg, avoiding contact with your shinbone. The tibialis is tight on most people, particularly if you walk fast. A tube of similar length and width like PVC conduit can also be used. Place a cushion behind you for comfort.

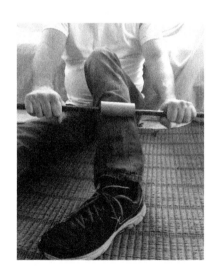

L15 Ant tib cross grip

This Self Massage technique for the anterior tibialis requires reasonable hand strength and a degree of knee flexibility too. Rest one ankle up on your other knee. Hook the fingertips of one hand into the muscle and use the other hand to guide and strengthen a back and forth motion across the muscle. People are often surprised how sensitive the ant tibs can be under even moderate pressure, so use whatever force you can relax into.

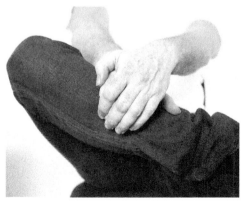

People who walk fast get tight in the ant tibs. There are pressure points along this muscle, which you will find in the chapter *Self Acupressure and Shiatsu.*

L16 Gentle rub

If you are elderly, sensitive or weak, Self Massage can be applied with light stroking. This helps the circulation in your skin. The feet and lower legs are usually the first parts of the body to suffer from poor circulation. If your feet swell, feel numb or sore, or are starting to darken, they will become more susceptible to infection and will heal more slowly.

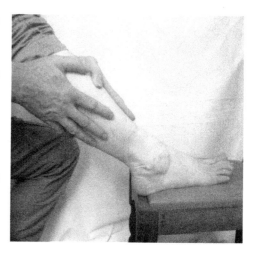

Always stroke upward, being careful to avoid any broken or delicate skin or varicose veins. You may be surprised at how much better this gentle technique can help you feel.

If you have trouble reaching down far enough, a long-handled dermal brush is an inexpensive massage tool that you can use for this. It is much easier to gently rub your feet and back with the long handle.

You can moisturise your skin as you do this. Placing your foot up on a chair in front of you can make gentle rubbing of your feet and calves easier.

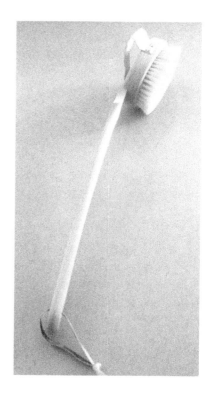

You can use dermal brushing on your arms and body too. Gentle rub is a softer technique than the others shown so far but it could be just what you need.

When we feel strong and robust it is easier to enjoy firmer massage but when we are in a weakened or emotionally fragile state, gentle is often better.

The "cuddle hormone" oxytocin is stimulated when your skin is lightly caressed, so there are emotional benefits as well as physical ones.

The act of giving yourself a dermal brush Self Massage all over your body can also give your shoulders and arms good stretching exercise.

14.3 LEG TECHNIQUES FOR BIGGER BODIES

Some of the Self Massage techniques in this chapter are difficult for anybody with a large abdomen because of difficulty with reaching the lower legs. Using a walking stick effectively enables you to reach around your abdomen, so this group of techniques is illustrated with a large-bellied model.

People who are overweight often have knee pain because of the extra downward pressure on the knee joint and because the legs have to work harder to carry them. If you are one of these people, the following techniques may help you. Ensure your stick has no sharp or rough edges. **Do not massage over varicose veins**.

Please note: umbrellas are unsuitable for these exercises and should not be used.

L17 One calf stick

Place the walking stick behind one calf and grasp both ends. Lean forward and back to apply pressure to the back of the calf in an up and down motion. Apply more pressure when sliding upward than downward, to assist blood flow. If you feel that one calf or knee is more painful than the other, you can focus your attention on that side. Placing a tube around your stick as in **L12 Peroneus roll** and **L14 Tibial roll** (pages 135 and 136) can help make this easier to apply.

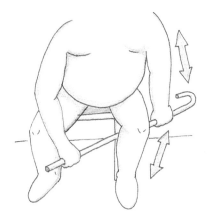

If you are fairly short and your own walking stick is too short to get good leverage, use a longer stick.

L18 Double calf stick

While seated, grasp both ends of your walking stick and hold it sideways behind your calves. Push it forward against your calves and slide it up and down against the muscle. It is best if the up stroke is firmer than the down stroke.

Some knee pain is muscular in origin, and this technique can help alleviate such knee pain.

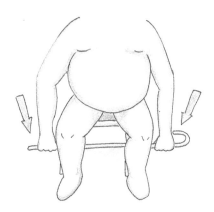

L19 One thigh stick

Press your walking stick down against one thigh, using the other hand to hold the stick steady against your opposite thigh. Use a comfortable amount of pressure as you move the stick up and down the thigh. It is best that the up stroke be a bit stronger than the down stroke. Placing a tube around your stick as in **L12 Peroneus roll** and **L14 Tibial roll** (pages 135 and 136) can help make this easier to apply.

Tightness in these muscles makes it harder to climb stairs and can produce hip and knee pain.

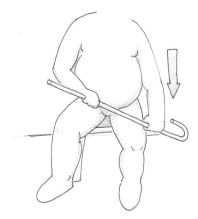

L20 Two thigh stick

Grasping both ends of the walking stick, press down and slide it back and forth to relieve muscular tension in the front of your thigh. Both thighs are done at once. Apply firm but comfortable pressure. The stroke toward your body should be slightly firmer than the away stroke.

When these muscles get tight, raising your legs to climb ladders and stairs becomes more difficult.

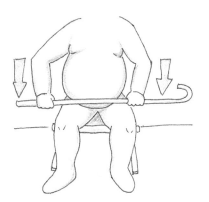

L21 Inner thigh press

Rest a walking stick on your thigh, then press and slide the end of the curved handle along your inner thigh. Massaging pressure is created by pulling the stick away to the side with one hand and pushing the curved handle against your inner thigh with the other.

You may be surprised at how even moderate pressure can produce a strong sensation. Use whatever pressure you desire and relax into it while breathing out. This can relieve knee pain.

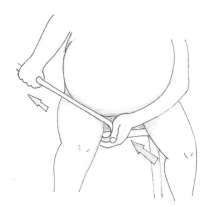

L22 Hamstring stick

You will need to sit a bit closer to the edge of your seat for this one. Rest one end of the stick on the top of one thigh and place the other end beneath the other thigh. Steady the upper end of the stick with one hand and with the other, pull the lower end of the stick firmly upward and toward your body in order to apply a good firm massaging pressure to your hamstrings. Placing a tube around your stick as in **L12 Peroneus roll** and **L14 Tibial roll** (pages 135 and 136) can help make this easier to apply.

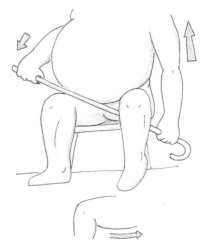

Some find this is a little ticklish to start with, so experiment with the pressure and tempo. Exhaling as you apply pressure can help you relax into it.

L23 Side handle

This exercise targets the hip abductors on the outside of your thigh. Press the end of the walking stick handle firmly against your outer thigh and slide it up and down. Make the stroke up toward your hip firmer than the stroke down toward your knee. You can increase the pressure by pulling the walking stick with your other hand.

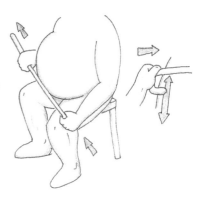

The hip abductors can produce hip and knee pain when they get stiff.

L24 Calf probe

Use the end of your walking stick to locate and Self Massage stiff inner calf and foot muscles. This includes the muscle on your foot's inner edge beneath your inner anklebone (malleolus). Press and hold on each stiff muscle for at least 20 seconds.

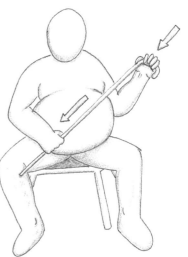

The muscle below the inner anklebone can get very stiff and usually responds well to massage.

The foot muscles indicated in the diagram here get stiff with dropped foot arches.

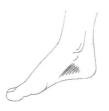

14.4 EXERCISES FOR THE FEET AND LEGS

L25 Backward toe stretch

Stretching your toes backward can sooth the tough fibrous fascia layer that is under the skin of your soles. This tissue is present in your palms too, making these areas much more resistant to friction than the rest of your skin.

Stretch each and every individual toe backward as far as comfort allows, and hold the toe in that extended position for a minimum of 20 seconds.

If the balls of your feet get sore, you should do this often.

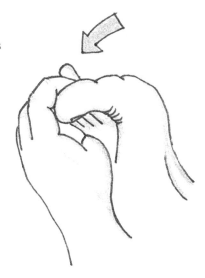

L26 Forward toe stretch

This is the opposite of **L25 Backward toe stretch**. Bend each of your toes forward as far as possible, ensuring that each and every toe joint bends. Elderly people often have stiff toe joints that can make walking uncomfortable. This exercise can help prevent toe problems and perhaps even fix an existing stiff toe.

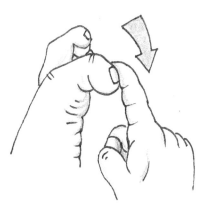

If you have trouble reaching your feet and cannot convince anybody else to do it for you, try stretching your toes back and forth against a cushion placed on the floor in front of your chair.

L27 Dry sand walking stretch/strength

Walking in dry sand is an excellent stretch for your toes and a good strength exercise for the muscles in the sole of your foot.

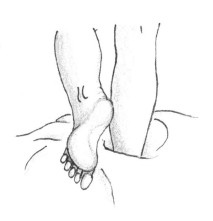

If you neither live nor work near a beach, you can still dry sand walk in a children's sandpit. Please be mindful of sharp objects hidden from view in the sand. Run a rake over the sand first if you can.

L28 Toe pickup flex

Use your toes to pick up small objects like tissue paper from the floor. Doing this often will help strengthen the arches of your feet. Having good foot strength and dexterity is good for your balance too.

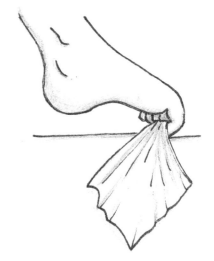

L29 Random foot roll

Position a cylindrical object like a drink can or full water bottle under one foot. Start by rolling it up and down along your foot, and then start to roll it sideways and diagonally, controlling its direction with ankle and foot movements. Use your foot and lower leg muscles to control its movement while frequently changing direction. You can do this sitting up or lying on your back with your knees bent.

This is a Self Massage as well as an exercise, particularly if you do it with a bumpy plastic bottle.

Dr. Bushman's exercises **M1 Tube pick up** and **M3 Sock stand** (page 45) in the Functional Fitness chapter are also good for strengthening foot muscles.

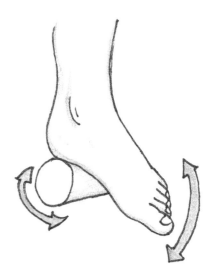

There are numerous small muscles in the soles of your feet, which get lazy from walking only on flat level surfaces. This can affect your balance and sure-footedness. These exercises will help restore strength to these muscles and improve your functional fitness.

L30 Ankle bend flex

For this exercise you will need an exercise band such as a Thera-Band, fastened to something low and solid like a couch leg.

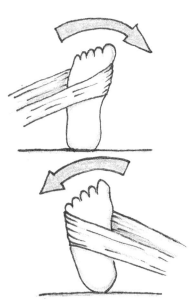

Sit on a chair and place your foot in the band, as shown at right. Roll your foot sideways on your heel in a motion like a windshield wiper. It is important that the strength of the band matches the strength of your ankles, so use a weaker Thera-Band if you are struggling.

These exercises may help prevent you rolling over on your ankle when you walk or run.

Do both directions to strengthen both sides of the ankle.

L31 Static ankle flex

If you have no exercise bands, pressing your foot sideways against your desk at work can give you a similar benefit.

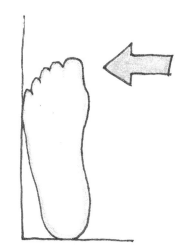

If you remember to be resourceful with your time you can fit a lot more exercise in. It's a matter of keeping your eyes open for the opportunities.

It is worth remembering too that wiggling your toes is good for your circulation. This exercise will also help your circulation.

L32 Wobble board balance

Wobble boards are marketed by different names, but the idea is the same. Fortunately you can buy these cheaply in department stores now. Hold onto something steady if you need to. Wobble boards utilize calf as well as foot muscles and can improve your balance.

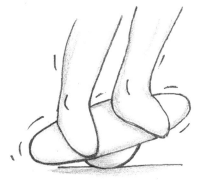

L33 Heel raises

Stand on a slightly raised ledge so that your toes are higher than your heels. With both feet, raise and lower your body onto the balls of your feet. Do as many reps as you are able.

If this is too hard for you, you can still do heel raises on a flat floor (without the ledge). Or, to make this exercise more challenging, heel raise on one foot at a time.

If you have a damaged Achilles tendon, do not do this exercise.

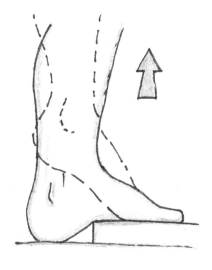

L34 Band toe up flex

To strengthen the ant tibs on the front of your shins, fasten the ends of a Thera-Band to something solid like a couch leg. Sit on a chair, place your foot into the band loop and flex your toes up toward you. Do both sides.

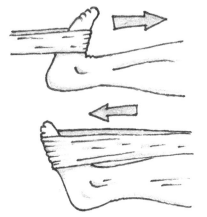

L35 Band toe down flex

To strengthen your calves, sit on a chair and hold the ends of the Thera-Bands in your hands. Point your toes downward away from your body. Do both sides.

L36 Ball squats

Ball squats are an effective isometric exercise to strengthen your knees. Do not bend your knees more acutely than 90 degrees if it hurts them. Hold this position as long as you can. Lean back against the ball for greater comfort.

Old knee injuries often cause arthritis later in life. If squatting is painful even after Self Massage, squat no lower than comfort allows.

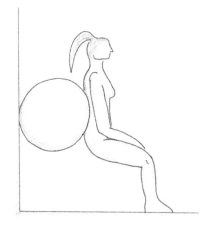

L37 Lateral quad stretch

Lie on your side on the floor or on a firm bed. Bend your top leg backward from the knee and pull it backward with your hand as far as comfort allows. You will feel a stretch in the front of your thigh that you should maintain for a minimum of 20 seconds. Do both sides.

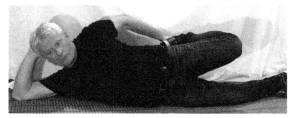

This stretch will work on your quads and your shin muscles at the same time. While it can be done in the standing position, this way is safer and more effective because it is easier to relax into the stretch.

L38 Seated hamstring stretch

Sit on the floor or a firm bed with one leg outstretched in front of you. Reach down to pull your toes back with one hand while straightening your leg with pressure on the thigh above the knee with your other. Breathe out as you stretch. If you cannot reach your toes, use a towel or belt looped around the ball of your foot to pull your toes toward your body (this will stretch your calves too). Hold for 20 seconds and then do the other side.

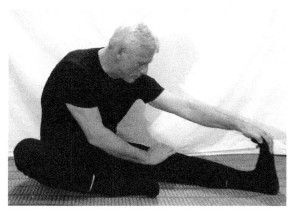

L39 Standing calf stretch

With legs straight, stand facing a wall and place the ball of one foot against the wall with your heel on the floor. With your other foot slightly behind you, raise its heel and lean forward. This will stretch the back of the forward leg. Hold the stretch for 20 seconds and then do the other side.

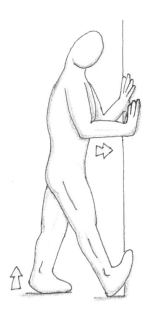

Steady your balance with your hands on the wall if you need to. If your calves are flexible there is a lower chance of tearing them or the Achilles tendon they attach to.

This is a good handy stretch you can do almost anywhere.

L40 Abductor leg raises

Lie on your side and raise your upper leg directly sideways (upward). Hold this position for as long as you can. Note that this exercise is more difficult than it looks. Lie on the floor in front of a mirror to ensure your hips and shoulders are in a straight line with one another.

Do a few reps each side. Pad your elbow if the floor is a bit hard.

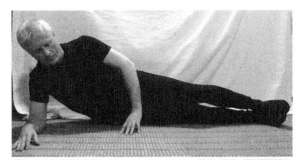

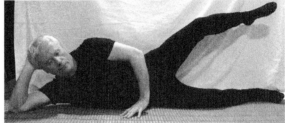

L41 Adductor leg raises

Lie on your side propped up on your elbow. Place the foot of the upper leg in front of the knee of the straightened lower leg, then raise your lower leg upward. Hold this position for as long as comfort allows.

This exercise strengthens your inner thigh muscles. Do both sides.

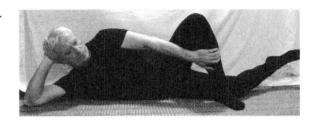

Note: it is important that the foot of the upper leg be placed **in front of** the straightened lower leg. This ensures that the adductor muscle is targeted. If done correctly, you will feel the effort in the inner thigh of the lower leg.

Your adductors and abductors play an important role in the alignment of your legs when you run and walk, so they are worth exercising.

These exercises tend to be more popular with women than men because of their reputation for firming the butt and thighs. While they are undoubtedly good for leg strength, the elimination of cellulite cannot be directly addressed by leg raises. A wider strategy is required.

You do not need weights to strengthen your hip muscles – the weight of your own leg is all the resistance you need.

L42 Lateral leg stretch

Kneel on the floor or on a cushion for comfort. Straighten one leg out sideways to stretch the adductors on the inside of your thigh. Slowly ease yourself into this position until you feel the adductors stretching, and hold it for 20 to 30 seconds.

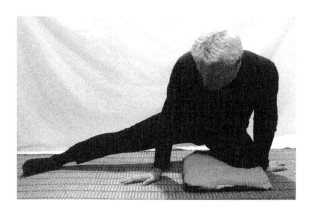

If this hurts your knee or thigh, stop at once. This stretch should not be painful but there might be mild discomfort. If you cannot kneel, lean on a table and do this standing.

L43 Supine adductor stretch

Lie down on your back and place your heels together, knees bent and pointing outward. Relax and let your knees slowly fall toward the floor. If you are unable to relax them fully sideways, it is OK to wedge equal sized pillows beneath the sides of your legs. Relax into the stretch for 30 seconds.

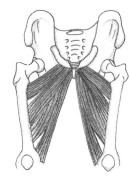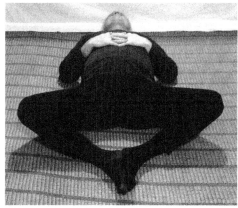

L44 Seated adductor stretch

Sit on your floor, on a cushion, or on a firm bed. Place the soles of your feet together and push downward on your knees with a firm constant pressure for 20 to 30 seconds. Do **not** use a rocking or bouncing motion for this exercise.

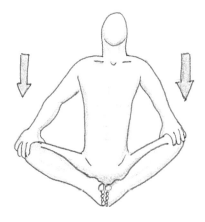

As with many of the Self Massage techniques and exercises in this book, you can do this at home while watching the TV. Go easy to start with.

L45 Lunge stretch/strength

With hand weights held by your side, step across the room with exaggerated long strides to strengthen your thighs. Your strides should be long enough that the ankle of the front leg remains slightly in front of the knee. Keep your back straight at all times.

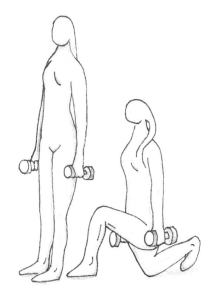

Many people like to do this exercise with a barbell across their shoulders. If you insist on using the barbell on your shoulders, get someone who knows how to do it properly to show you so you can avoid injury, as the bar can push your head and neck forward. Note that this is a leg exercise, not an upper back one.

Wearing a weighted vest for lunges is another way to increase your working load.

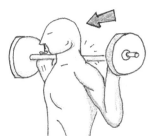

If it is easier to stride further ahead with one leg more than the other, you may have some stiffness in your hips or calves that Self Massage should be applied to.

If your knees twinge doing this exercise, stop.

L46 Supine hamstring stretch

Lie flat on your back, and loop a belt or towel around the ball of your foot. Pull back on your raised straightened leg to improve your hamstring flexibility. This exercise is useful if the muscles at the back of your legs are so tight that you cannot touch your toes.

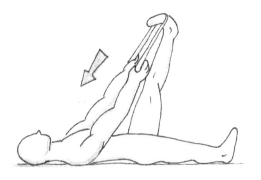

Your upper back gets some exercise with this too.

14.5 ADDITIONAL EXERCISES

A number of exercises covered in earlier chapters, in particular Lower Body, are also great leg exercises. These stretches help both your legs and lower body.

B21 Standing groin stretch

This exercise stretches your hip flexors and your calf. Keep your heels on the floor, ease into position and exhale. Hold this position for at least 20 seconds. It should look and feel a bit like Tai Chi.

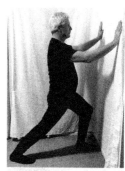

B19 Pigeon stretch

This exercise stretches the abductors on the outside of the thigh, in addition to the butt muscles (gluteals). The stretch should be felt from your knee to your hip. Hold the stretch for 20 seconds, then do the other side.

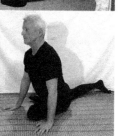

B23 Knee to ankle butt stretch

This stretch and others similar to it are good at simultaneously stretching your butt, thigh and calf muscles. This exercise is one of the more difficult stretches in this book.

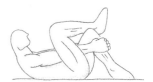

B20 Standing butt stretch

This is a good stretch for your thigh and butt muscles. Benches and desks of sound structure and appropriate height can be used. This stretch can relieve back pain and sciatica. Leaning forward will lengthen and intensify the stretch.

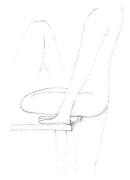

There are more leg exercises in the Functional Fitness chapter.

14.6 RISKY LEG AND FEET EXERCISES

Leg raises can be very tough on the end play movement of the knees, the last 10 degrees in particular.

Maybe you have done these before without any incident but as knee cartilage thins and scar tissue increases, this exercise is more likely to injure your knees.

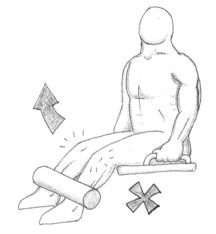

Leg press can stir up old knee and back trauma if you even slightly lose form and overdo it. I have known several otherwise intelligent men who have been injured in impromptu strength tests with their friends in gyms on the leg press.

The heavy weights on this apparatus act like a lightning rod for competitive male behavior. I have known people who have needed surgery for the after-effects of this.

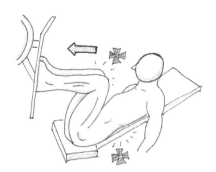

150

PART III

Advanced techniques and branching out.

15 ADVANCED SELF MASSAGE

The Self Massage techniques in this chapter apply more pressure to your muscles than the techniques presented in Part II of this book. **If the softer techniques were too painful to do then the advanced ones that follow will be way too much for you.**

If you have osteoporosis, seek advice from your doctor and show them this book before you do advanced Self Massage.

X1 Supine neck ball

If the Self Massage techniques in the Neck & Jaw chapter have not sufficiently loosened your neck muscles, try this technique. Lie supine with two tennis balls under the top of your neck immediately below your skull.

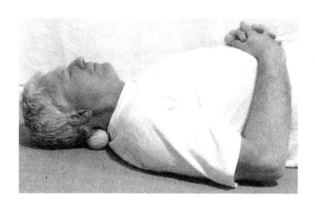

This can be effective in helping you sleep better and help ease and prevent headaches. Try not to fall asleep in this position, because you will wake up some time later feeling like you were on the balls for too long.

If you get drowsy, you have had enough.

X2 Neck stick

Lie on your back with your arms in the surrender position and with your walking stick across your hands and the stick across the top of your neck. Relax into the pressure. Wrap a towel around the stick if it feels too hard. Stop if this hurts or if you feel sleepy, dizzy or nauseous.

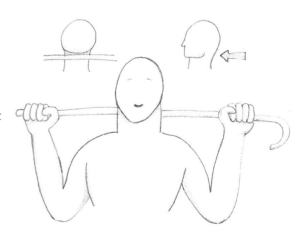

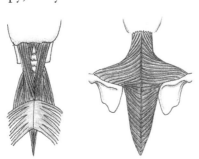

X3   Upper back floor balls

If you have already tried **S3** to **S7** (pages 75 to 77) and found them comfortable, this technique can be used to apply more pressure to your back. It is performed supine (on your back) on the floor or a firm mattress. Position two balls of equal firmness on either side of the spine, at the same level. Work the balls up and down along the back muscles, from below your neck to the level of the lowest rib.

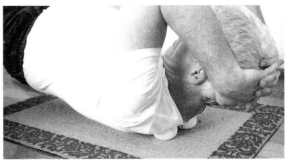

To create extra pressure over the tennis balls, press down with your heels against the floor and raise your butt a few inches. The more the balls support your body weight, the firmer the massage. Try softer balls first before moving to harder ones.

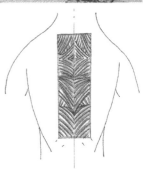

You might hear and feel some harmless pleasant popping sensations as you do this, but if you feel pain, cease immediately.

X4   Supine floor roll

This technique uses a foam roller and your body weight to apply pressure to the muscles of the back. Place your hands behind your head, bend your legs and use your heels to lift your butt off the floor. Roll back and forth on the roller slowly from shoulder level to your lower back. This can feel a bit intense to start with, in which case you can wear a thick pullover or wrap the roller in a small towel. Stop if it hurts.

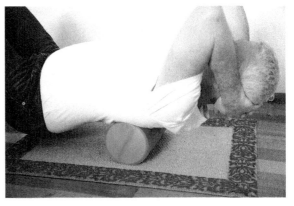

Do this technique after you have already tried **S3** to **S7** (pages 75 to 77) against the wall without any difficulty.

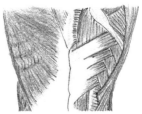

X5   Supine shoulder roll

If you have tried **S3 Shoulder blade wall roll** and **S4 Upper back wall roll** (page 75) with a firm ball and found after a few minutes of using those techniques that you would like to apply deeper pressure, try this technique.

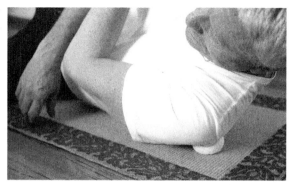

Lie on your back at about a 45-degree angle and with a tennis ball directly under your shoulder blade. Move the ball slowly to find the pressure points. This can be just what you need after a day in front of the computer – the mouse can really tense these muscles up.

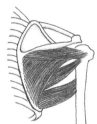

You are aiming for the thickest part of the muscle. Do not roll over the bony ridges of the shoulder blade.

If this gets painful, stop at once.

X6   Shoulder floor roll

This is a stronger version of **S2 Shoulder wall roll, S9 Shoulder corner press**, and **S10 Chest plunger press** (pages 74 and 78). Try this one if you have already tried those techniques and you want deeper pressure. Lie face down so that the tennis ball is moving under the front of your shoulder and on the top of your chest.

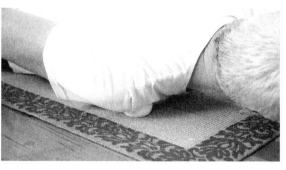

These muscles do a lot of work. Each time you reach forward and across your body these muscles engage.

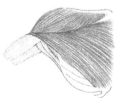

If you like doing push-ups and bench presses you need to Self Massage these muscles. They can get surprisingly tight.

X7 Floor lat roll

Foam rolling your lats can be performed lying sideways. Roll along the side of your rib cage from your shoulder down. If you had difficulty relaxing into **S31 Lat wall stretch** (page 91), this will probably be too painful to relax into. You may need to wrap a small fluffy towel around the roller to begin with. If you swim a lot, these muscles need Self Massaging.

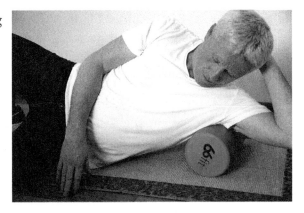

X8 Prone hip roll

Foam rolling your thigh muscles massages and stretches them at the same time. Position yourself on the floor with one leg outstretched backward and the other forward (in a low crawling posture). Lower yourself even further so that you can roll the entire length of your front thigh muscles (quadriceps) on the foam roller. Work the roller back and forth several times along your quads and stop when you have had enough, or if it hurts. If your hips are quite stiff, you may struggle to relax into this position. If it is a struggle, stop.

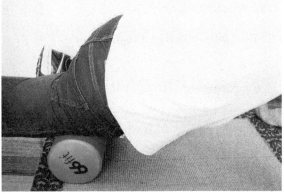

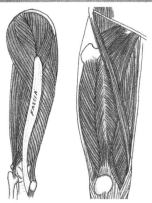

This is another strong technique that can be difficult to relax into, so breathe out as you do it.

If you have a sit down job and can relax into the pressure, you should regularly do this technique to keep your hip muscles supple.

X9   Lateral floor press

If you have tried **B1** to **B4** (pages 115 and 116) and you felt some release of muscle tension but not as much as desired, try this technique. Lie on your side and locate the tennis ball in the gap at your side above your hip but below your ribs. You are pressuring the same point as **B4 Lumbar wall lean** (page 116), but lying relaxed into it.

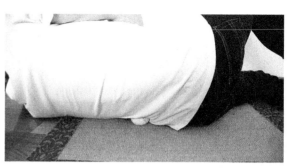

If you have just injured your back, don't do this technique.

This band of muscle next to your spine has three more superficial layers of abdominal muscle above it. If you find bending sideways at your waist difficult or you get lower back pain from time to time and sit down a lot, you should try to Self Massage these muscles.

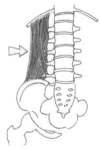

X10 Plunger wall press

If you coped with **X9 Lateral floor press**, try this technique. Stick the suction cup at waist height onto a smooth wall. Standing side-on to the wall, hold the plunger handle firmly and position the tip of the handle between the top of the hip and the lowest rib. (Do **not** press on the rib.)

With your feet widely spaced for good balance, gradually ease your weight onto the plunger to apply pressure. **This is not supposed to hurt – if it does, stop doing it or ease off**. Do not rock into this, just ease in for 20 seconds then ease off.

The floor on which you are standing needs to have thoroughly good traction so you do not slip while attempting this. Be balanced and stay fully focused on what you are doing, and **don't let go until you finish**.

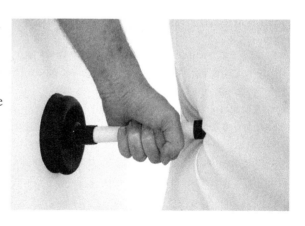

This is the deepest Self Massage technique for your lower back in this book.

157

X11 Lumbar roll

Locate two tennis balls on either side of your lower back over the thickest parts of the muscle. When they are properly in place, ease your weight down onto them. Press down with your heels and move your body slowly back and forth over the balls. If you find a position particularly relaxing, lie on that point a bit longer. The balls should rest over muscle, not over bone. Only do this if the softer techniques were too mild. If it hurts, stop doing it.

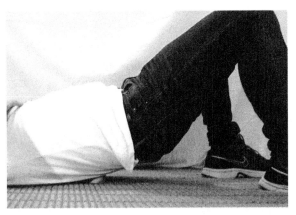

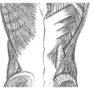

Try the techniques **B1 Lumbar rub**, **B2 Lumbar knuckles**, and **B3 Seated lumbar knuckles** (page 115) first, and use softer balls to start with.

Keep the balls at the same level on either side of the spine.

X12 Lateral hip roll

Lie on your side and place a ball between the bony bumps on your side – the pelvic arch at the top and the hip bump about six inches lower down. Tip yourself slightly back and forth from your hips so the ball Self Massages you from your buttock toward your groin and back again. Move your body to find the best massage spots. If it hurts, stop.

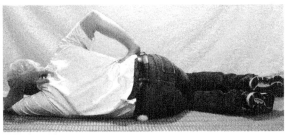

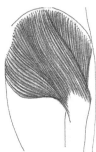

X13 Hip floor roll

There are some large strong muscles located beneath the side arch of your pelvis and above the bump of bone just below it. Stiffness here restricts normal movement, distorts your posture, and causes back and hip pain. Lie on your back on the floor or a firm mattress and place a ball of sufficient firmness under each buttock. Each ball must be located in the same place under each muscle. Roll your body from side to side and up and down or just stay still if it feels good. If this hurts at all, stop.

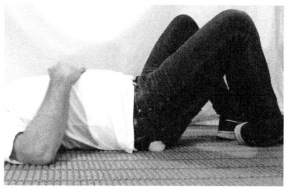

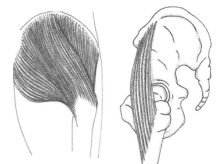

Stretch these muscles after 5 minutes of doing this technique.

X14 Supine buttock roll

If one buttock is particularly stiff and you would like to focus on loosening it, lie on your back with one ball under the thickest part of your butt muscle. Raise your knee on that side slowly up and down sideways onto the ball. This technique is similar to **X13** except that one ball is used instead of two.

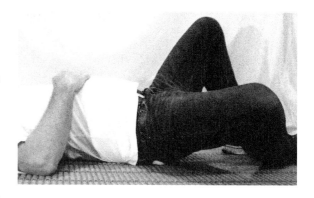

This can feel surprisingly sensitive the first time you try it so go lightly with a softer ball to start with. This technique can assist in the relief of sciatica.

X15 Lateral thigh roll

Lie on your side with the foam roller under your inner thigh. By turning back and forth from your hips you can Self Massage your adductors. This can help improve the flexibility of your inner thighs and relieve some types of knee and lower back pain.

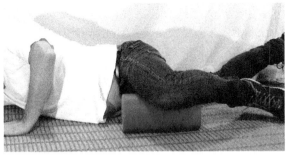

As with the other techniques in this chapter, you may be surprised how tight and sensitive these muscles are to pressure.

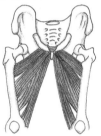

If you play a sport that requires kicking or sidestepping or if you do yoga, you need to add this technique to your training regime.

X16 Seated thigh roll

This technique simultaneously stretches and Self Massages your hamstrings. Sit on the floor and reach for your toes. If your hamstrings are too stiff to allow this, loop a belt or towel around the ball of your foot and pull the ends with your hands so the muscles behind your leg stretch. Place a ball under your thigh as you do this – this will Self Massage your hamstrings and stretch them at the same time. Hold for about 20 seconds and then do the other side.

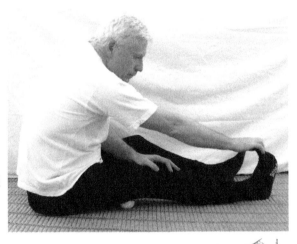

You can also apply downward pressure with one hand on the lower thigh (but never on top of the kneecap).

If you run a lot, doing this can help with muscle recovery after exercise.

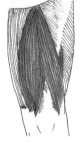

16 PERCUSSIVE SELF MASSAGE

Rather than slow rubbing, rolling and static pressure, percussive massage is like playing a drum, where that drum is you.

In Swedish massage, percussive techniques like chopping, pounding and cupping are collectively referred to as *tapotement*, in contrast to the smooth flowing *effleurage* strokes that are intended to sooth and relax. Tapotement can soften stiff muscles as well as effleurage can, but it is a far more stimulating and invigorating massage. Percussive Self Massage has a stimulating rather than sedating effect on the nervous system, which is why tapotement massage is used in pre-sport warm-ups. Stimulating massage improves alertness and vigor.

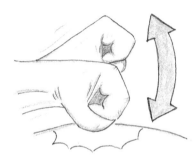

Percussive Self Massage is something you will often see people do as a tai chi warm-up. Chinese athletes use it before competing. You too can use it before you exercise. It can be especially useful as a warm-up on a cold day.

Even if you are not intending to do something strenuous, percussive Self Massage can help wake you up and focus your attention.

Like the other Self Massage techniques, you are in control of how deeply you work and how much pressure you apply to your own body. Once you find the best tempo and pressure for yourself, it will feel good, both during and afterward.

The key to doing good percussive or tapotement massage is to keep your wrists and elbows loose and moving as you go. Your hand/fist is rhythmically flapping back and forth as you make contact with the target muscles. The movement is initiated from the shoulder in a rippling flowing arm action. Once you find a rhythm, it is surprisingly easy, like playing bongo drums.

The first thing to do is to loosen your arms up – loosely wave your arms around by your sides for a few minutes so your wrists and elbows are lithe and ready to be used as free-moving hinges.

There are several surfaces of your hand that you can use for percussive Self Massage: pounding downward with the side of your fist; holding your fingertips together to concentrate contact for smaller areas such as the tops of your shoulders; as though you are knocking at a door; pounding upward with the thumb side of your fist; and slapping with your palm.

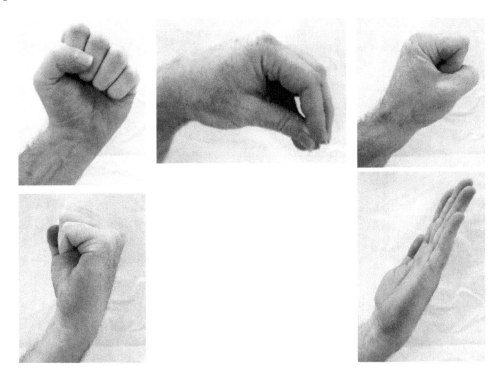

Like doing cardio exercise, percussive Self Massage is about finding a rhythm. Once you find a rhythm you can maintain, you can do percussive Self Massage for 10, 20 or even 30 minutes at a time if you wish.

Always remember to let your hands flick down from loose wrists. Do not hold your wrists or elbows in a rigid position or you will get tired very quickly. You do not need to use even pressure with both hands – in fact, it is easier to sustain a rhythm with uneven pressure. Practice on your thighs.

P1 Arm pound

Relax your massaged arm as you use a downward pounding stroke on it. Hold the wrist of the massaging arm loose as you flick your fist against your arm, as hard or as soft as you like. Continue right up to your chest. Then turn your palm down and do the other side of your arm.

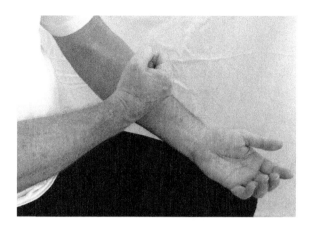

P2 Side pound

Hold onto one shoulder, and use the upper side of one fist to massage the back of the opposite upper arm with an upward motion. Angle your index knuckle upward for increased pressure. Do both arms.

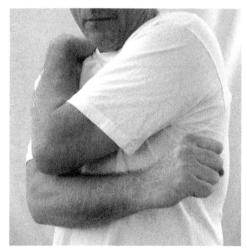

P3 Shoulder peck

Bunch your fingertips together and employ a flicking up and down stroke from your wrist to Self Massage your upper trapezius. You can use this stroke on your chest and shoulders too.

Go easy near your neck. Do not apply percussive Self Massage directly to your neck.

You can do this for longer if you rest the elbow of your massaging arm on a desk in front of you.

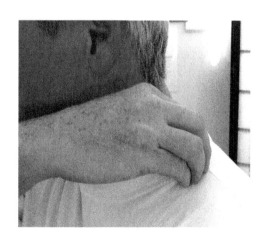

P4   Thigh pound

There is no need to tapote your belly, go straight to your thighs now. While sitting, pound your thighs at the front and sides, using different surfaces of your hands for different parts of your thigh.

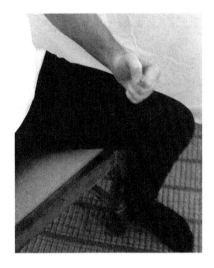

P5   Upward leg pound

Sit down and lift one foot onto another chair. Lean forward slightly and pound upward to percuss your hamstrings. You are unlikely to hurt yourself doing this so don't be timid about the pressure unless it hurts.

You can percussively Self Massage your calf from this position too.

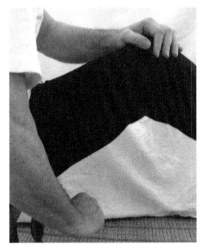

P6   Lower leg pound

With your foot placed on a chair, start knocking and pecking at those hard working muscles on the front and outside of your lower leg. Start low on the leg and work upward, being careful to avoid the bones.

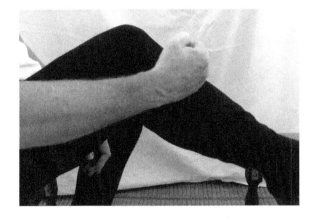

P7   Hip pound

While standing, pound around your hips, at the front, the sides, and on your butt muscles (using the thumb side of your fist). Do both hips at once. Create your own rhythm.

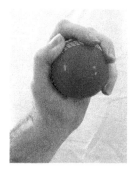 If you have a fairly tough body or sensitive hands, you can use a ball instead of your hands. You should start with a softer ball, but a harder ball like a baseball or cricket ball can be used once you are comfortable with the technique. As with any other type of massage, avoid contact with bone. Massage is for muscles.

Start with light pressure and keep your mind on what you are doing.

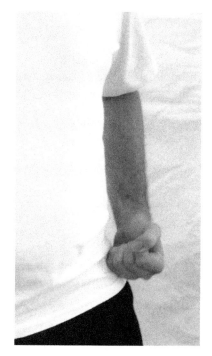

P8   Chest pound

Percussive Self Massage to the chest can help loosen chest congestion. Do not strike breast tissue – women should concentrate on the side and upper part of the rib cage.

Smoking and even just breathing in polluted air can congest your airways, as surely as a cold will. Use an open hand light smacking motion to begin with and then use a closed fist when you are comfortable with it.

If you are slight and frail, use a gentle force with these percussive techniques and try different parts of your hand to strike yourself with to find what is best for you.

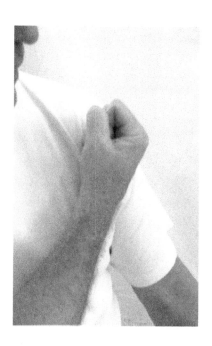

P9   Two hand pound

I find percussive Self Massage most useful on the larger muscles. With practice you can drum away rapidly using both hands on the big muscles of your chest, shoulders, hips and thighs. Remember that Self Massage should feel good, so alter your pressure and tempo if it doesn't.

The two handed drumming action of Percussive Self Massage also assists right and left brain crossover.

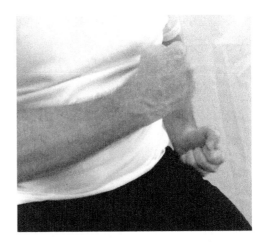

P10   Foot pound

Lift your ankle onto your knee and tap away with your knuckles onto the sole of your foot. It always felt good at the end of shiatsu classes when we did this. If your knee hurts, try resting your foot sideways on the chair in front of you.

Use your knuckles as shown or peck with your fingertips at your soles.

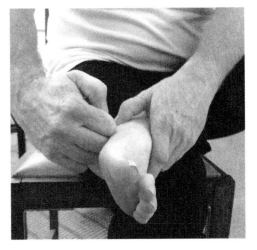

Always get your posture right and pay attention to what your body is telling you. If you have a neurological disease or injury, please show your physician this book before trying percussive Self Massage.

17 PRACTICAL POSTURAL TIPS

The illustrations and comments in this chapter are here to help you do simple everyday tasks more comfortably and easily. They will assist your functional fitness.

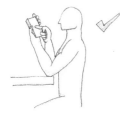

T1   Straight neck

Whether it is a book, a cell phone, or an iPad, raise the object so it is in front of your face and not at waist level.

Support your elbow to save your neck.

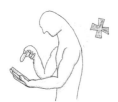

Your whole body is tipped forward when you hold even the lightest object in the manner shown in the lower illustration at left. This fatigues the muscles behind your neck and can cause headaches.

T2   Samurai pumpkin

When cutting something hard like a fresh pumpkin, it's an easy trap to fall into to seesaw the knife with your shoulders hunched up. Instead, brace your arms and place the heel of your hand on the blunt spine of the knife.

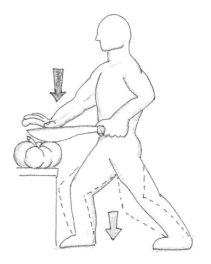

Keep your back straight and your arms braced, and drop your weight down by bending your knees. You will see how much easier and faster it is to cut your pumpkin. **Samurai swordsmen** are taught to lower their body in the same way to add power to a downward stroke.

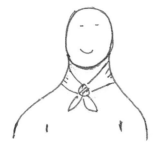

T3   Neck wrap

As we age, our necks often become more sensitive to cool breezes from indoor and outdoor sources. People get into the habit of unconsciously hunching to keep their neck covered. Try wearing a lightweight scarf if you get neck pain and see if it makes a difference to the comfort and posture of your neck. You may be surprised what a difference this makes to shoulder tension.

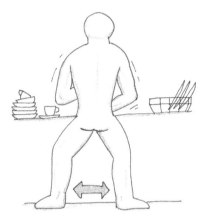

T4   Giraffe stance

If you are too tall for the work surface in front of you, don't lean over and bend your back. Instead, move your feet further apart like a giraffe at a water hole. This drops your center of gravity.

You can bend your knees slightly forward and brace them against the cupboard or bench in front of you for further stability if you like.

T5   Soldier stance

Soldiers use this trick on parade grounds to ease the pressure on their soles. Slowly shift your weight backward and forward and side to side; by doing so, the blood gets a chance to circulate better through your soles.

If you have a standing job, this can help make your feet a bit less uncomfortable at the day's end.

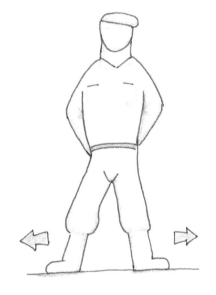

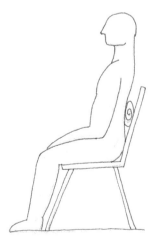

T6   Lumbar roll

Shown at left is an example typical of the cheap stackable seating you will find in school halls and many other places.

If you roll up a towel or a garment you can **support your lower back** better. It is much easier to pay attention to speakers when you are comfortably upright. It takes more effort for core muscles to support a crooked posture than a straight one. Better posture creates better balance and less muscle fatigue.

T7 Tai chi bench stance

Whether you are giving someone a massage, sawing plywood or shaping a surfboard, you will work with greater precision, strength and balance by moving your body to move your hands.

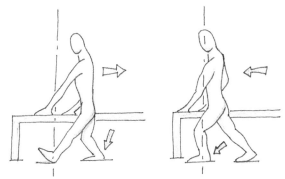

Move your body by shifting your weight from your back foot to your front foot and back again. Keep your back straight and your feet a good distance apart, as though you are alternating between front and back stance in karate. It is easier to apply downward pressure from directly above.

T8 Weeding stance

If you want to keep gardening for many more years, you should learn this posture to save your knees and back (see **M9 Bending down** on page 49). Your hamstrings, butt and calf muscles should feel like they are doing the work of holding your body up, not your back. **Do not bend your knees any more acutely than illustrated.**

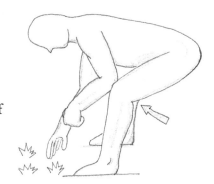

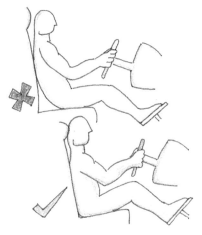

T9   Car seating

Give your car seat a chance to support your lower back properly.

Pull your butt back against the back of your seat and move your seat far enough forward that you can place either heel against the floor.

Then re-adjust your mirrors.

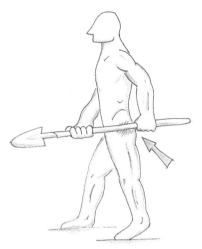

T10   Shovel hip

Try holding the middle of the shovel handle against your hip. Holding a load against your body makes it easier to carry. Your hip can be used as a fulcrum from this position.

Do not break contact between your hip and shovel handle and you may be surprised at how much easier shoveling becomes. Move your legs, not your arms, to shift the soil.

T11 Chest strap

Even a lightweight backpack will feel progressively heavier the longer you carry it. The chest strap that many backpacks are made with now is there to relieve tension on the front of your shoulders. These straps often go unused because some people think it looks "uncool." If you are a backpack user give it a try – not only is it easier on your shoulders, it is good for your posture too.

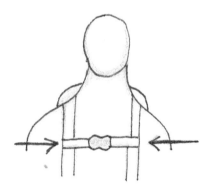

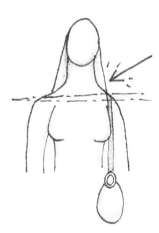

T12   Bag shoulder

If you are a handbag wearer, take turns carrying it on either shoulder. Your shoulder will always be hitched up slightly higher on the side you wear it on. Many women get a chronically tight neck and shoulder through carrying exclusively on one side. The same applies to laptop bags, clutches, briefcases and folders.

Don't forget to do regular neck stretches.

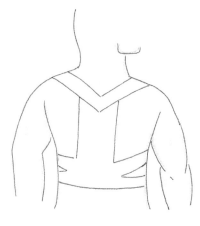

T13   Shoulder brace

There are various types of upper back braces that open your chest up and hold your shoulders back. They can make your posture look and feel better, but just remember that they are no substitute for strong postural muscles.

The best way of using these is to prove to yourself how much better good posture can make you look and feel. Use this as a motivation to do postural exercises to strengthen your back muscles so that you won't need to wear one. If you do not exercise the muscles of your upper back, wearing a brace might even make your back muscles lazy, weak and more injury prone.

T14 Knee lift

Lifting even light weights can hurt you if your lifting posture is poor.

Don't take shortcuts, even for small lifts and even if you are in a hurry. **Always adopt a good lifting posture from the start.** If you do not have the time to lift properly, finding the time to visit a chiropractor after you hurt your back will even be more difficult.

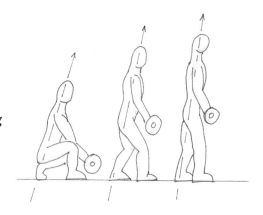

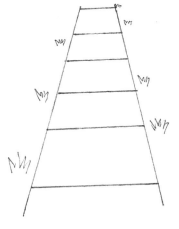

T15   Line step

The next time you walk along an evenly segmented path, take notice of where each foot makes contact. It is an easy way to see how even your stride is. If you find you are stepping with a shorter stride on one side, that leg may be slightly shorter than the other one and you may need to visit an orthotist or podiatrist for foot levelers.

Or you might have even leg lengths but have uneven muscular tone or flexibility in the hip or leg muscles, which Self Massage and stretching can help remediate. An even stride is good for your spine – **Line step** is an easy way to test it.

171

T16 Stand up desk

Standing instead of sitting at your workstation can give your lower back a welcome break. You will see best results if you stand straight with your feet sharing the weight evenly.

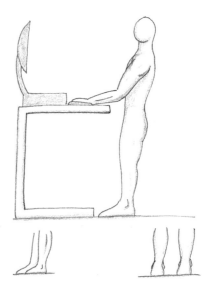

Place your feet a shoulder's width apart and constantly and slowly shift your weight from side to side. Alternate this with standing with one foot forward and the other back, slowly shifting your weight from front to back and then to the front again. Change sides regularly.

If you work seated part of the time and take little walk breaks, it can help make your body happier at the day's end. Make a point of periodically looking at distant objects to protect yourself against eyestrain.

Whether seated or standing, keep a straight back with your chin in, shoulders back and seat tipped forward.

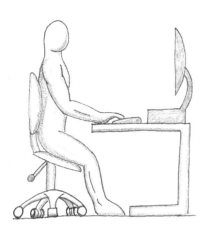

Imagine you are squeezing grapefruit between your shoulder blades numerous times through the day. Pulling your shoulders back helps you stay straight.

Stretching your chest and shoulders frequently also reduces muscle tension at the front of your body. Exercises **S18 Backward arm stretch** (page 83), **S20 Corner shoulder stretch** (page 85), **S21 Open chest stretch** (page 85), and **A12 Backward triceps stretch** (page 100) are useful for this.

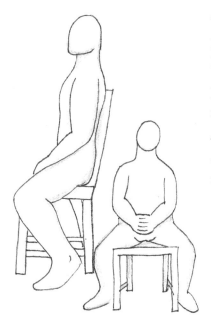

T17   Straddle chair

If you have to make do with poor seating, spread your knees as shown, as it can keep your back straighter.

Move your feet back below your hips and it will restore the normal curve to your lower back.

The chair will eventually create pressure on your inner thighs, but for short periods of time, this is a more posture-friendly way of using these older-style chairs.

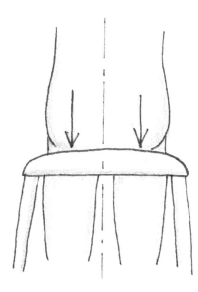

T18   Even butt

It is possible to be so used to sitting with a lean toward one side that we don't even realize it. Sit in front of a mirror and focus on feeling an even amount of pressure under each buttock. That pressure is the most reliable way of knowing if your spine is perpendicular. People are usually a bit shocked at how crooked they really are when trying this test. **Sitting on even a thin wallet tips you off center. It is not good for your back to sit with objects in your back pocket.**

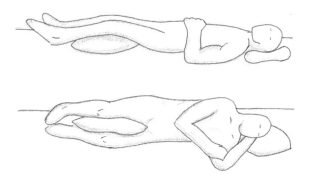

T19   Sleep pillows

Use pillows as shown to position your body for a better night's sleep. Nurses use such methods to make patients comfortable. If you struggle to get to sleep, try these.

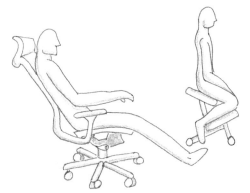

T20   Ergonomic seating

There is some innovative ergonomic office seating now available, designed to support better posture. Desks with adjustable height settings can be used with them to better suit our differing heights and proportions. If you spend a lot of time sitting, they are worth checking out.

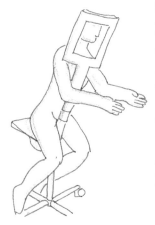

Swapping seating at intervals can also help keep you more comfortable for longer.

You can't really know what will work for you until you try. You can also alternate between being seated and standing up.

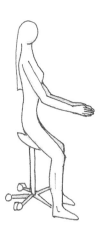

The ideal angle between thigh and torso for sitting is 135 degrees, which is one and a half right angles, not a right angle. Sometimes prospective buyers are put off by the lack of back support, but when your leg hangs lower you don't feel the need to lean back in your chair.

18 SELF MASSAGE & REFLEXOLOGY

Reflexology was used in ancient Egypt and China and was revived by physiotherapist Eunice Ingham and Dr. William Fitzgerald last century. Hand and foot reflexology is still enjoying renewed interest around the world. In 2005 it was reported that over 20% of the Danish population regularly used it.

Reflexology is one of the easier massage styles to learn and does not require the same amount of physical effort as whole body massage styles. The theory behind reflexology is that by palpating designated points around your hands and feet, other parts of your body can receive a benefit.

Not all reflexology charts are the same, so if you are already more familiar with charts that differ slightly from those shown here, by all means use them instead.

You can use your bare hands to do this or a massage tool such as the Thumbsaver.

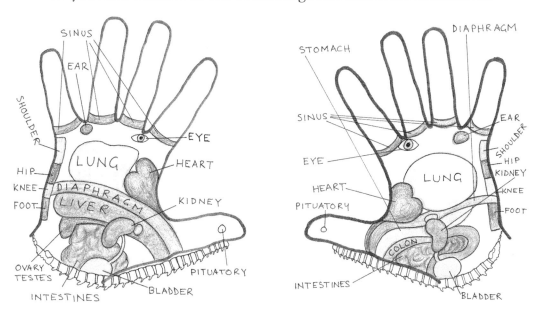

Foot reflexology is used in much the same way as hand reflexology. Like the hand charts, the foot charts on the next page might differ from other charts you have seen. Foot reflexology tends to be more popular than hand reflexology, perhaps because there are more people with sore feet than sore hands. I often kick my shoes off when at the computer and rub my aching feet with my toes and anklebones. It is an easy way to enjoy an improvised foot rub.

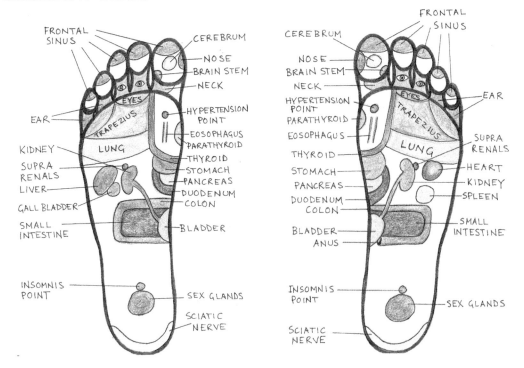

The foot reflexology chart at right is used in Zen shiatsu. In the other reflexology charts, the right and left feet and hands differ slightly from one another. With this chart, the feet are identical because they do not represent your internal organs but the three sections of your spine.

The lumbar spine (lower back) has 5 vertebrae (backbones), the lowest joining the sacrum (L5) and highest (L1) joining the thoracic spine.

The thoracic spine (mid-back) has 12 vertebrae. T12 joins the lower back and T1 at the top is attached to your cervical spine (neck). Your ribs are attached to your thoracic spine.

The cervical spine has 7 vertebrae. C7 joins the top of your thoracic spine and C1 at the top joins your skull. All vertebrae are numbered top to bottom.

If your back or neck is too sore to directly Self Massage, try using these reflexology points at the appropriate levels. Do both feet using whatever technique works best for you. For example, if your lower neck is sore rub over 6 & 7 on the neck line; for the lowest back pain, press 4 & 5 over the lower back line. Try it for yourself.

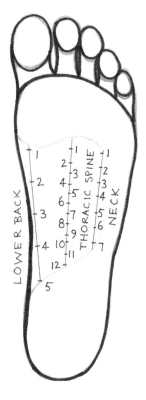

R1 Finger roll

Lightly grasp, roll and knead the sides of your fingers, starting with the reflexology sinus rings at their base and moving upward. Like all other forms of Self Massage, this should feel pleasant. Your sinus points are used here. This technique usually does make my sinuses feel clearer when I use it.

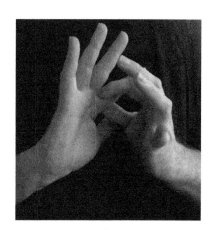

R2 Palm knuckles

Press your index knuckle all around the other palm, focusing on the softer areas between the bones and joints. This loosens muscles and fascia that tighten after strenuous use of your hands. Elderly Caucasian men are in a statistically high-risk group of suffering from hand contractures – this type of Self Massage (and stretching) might help you avoid your palms tightening up. Most hand reflexology points are used with this technique.

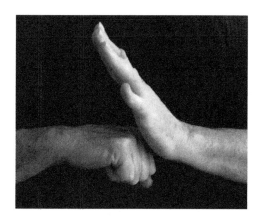

R3 Sole press

Your Thumbsaver is the tool of choice for finding the tender little spots on your soles. You can refer to the foot reflexology charts to see if there is a relationship between the chart and what you already know about your own body.

You can also do this to relieve the symptoms of plantar fasciitis (inflamed fascia on your soles). People in occupations that require a great deal of walking, like nurses and wait staff, need to take good care of their feet and this technique can help.

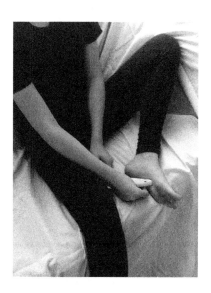

R4 Sole stick press

If you already have a need to carry a walking stick, why not turn it upside down when you are resting and Self Massage your soles. You do not have to pull the stick hard to feel good pressure.

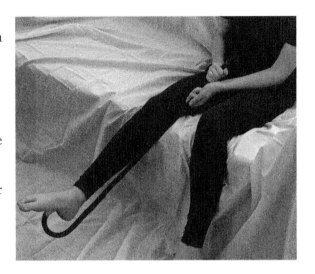

Please do not attempt this standing up, only while sitting. This is a great technique if you cannot easily reach your feet.

All foot reflexology points except for your toes can be reached this way.

R5 Standing sole press

If your knees are flexible, this is a good angle to apply easy downward pressure to your feet. Stand with your back to a sofa and rest your foot on the arm, then use your knuckles to Self Massage the arch of your foot. Keep your arm straight and lean slightly backward.

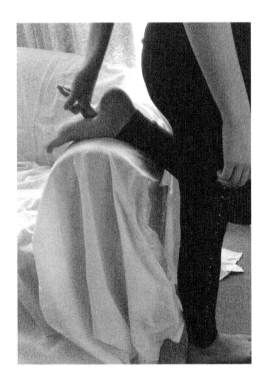

You can use your other hand to steady yourself against a doorway or wall, which is recommended when you try this for the first time.

To do this technique, your balance should be reasonably good. Your toes can also be Self Massaged with this technique.

19 SELF ACUPRESSURE & SHIATSU

Acupressure and shiatsu is applied to fingertip-sized areas over the muscles. These points on your skin have a slightly hollow feel to them because your skin surface tension is lower in those electronically detectable places.

Acupressure (Chinese) and Shiatsu (Japanese) are like acupuncture without the needles. These healing arts share similar origins and philosophies. Traditionally, acupressure and shiatsu points are pressed with your fingers and thumbs on other people, but it can be done on yourself, and massage tools can also be used. When using acupressure or shiatsu on yourself, a small massage tool like a Thumbsaver gives better-focused pressure and duration than your fingers alone can.

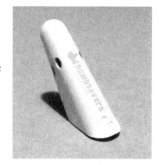

Acupressure and shiatsu are traditionally used for local muscle and joint problems and for the relief of internal problems like indigestion, period pain, asthma and cystitis. The theory behind these oriental therapies is too vast to abbreviate here but I invite you to locate these points on yourself and to apply a minute of pressure to each. Like other Self Massage, this should feel good, so see how it makes you feel.

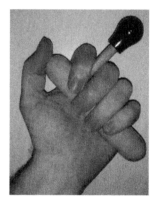

The Thumbsaver is a good massage tool to use on most acupressure and shiatsu points. A larger massage tool is stronger on calves.

C1 Leg to neck

These dots represent points on the gall bladder meridian, reputed to not only relieve calf, knee and ankle pain but also to help neck stiffness, headaches and sore eyes.

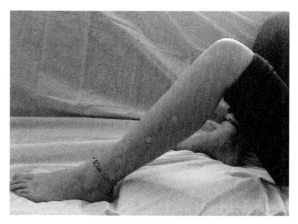

C2   Leg to belly

These highlighted points are located along the tibialis muscle next to your shinbone. People who walk fast get tight in these muscles. These pressure points are on the stomach meridian and are reputed to assist with abdominal pain, nausea and constipation.

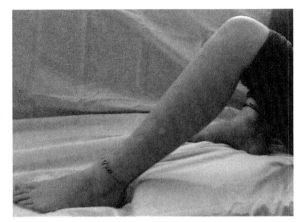

C3   Leg to groin

These spleen, liver and kidney points along the inner edge of the shin are reputed to relieve groin pain and dysmenorrhea and to help with infertility.

The soleus muscle lies under these points, which can be Self Massaged for the relief of shin splints. Thumbsavers are handy to use on these points. (See also **L6 Knuckle to calf** on page 133.)

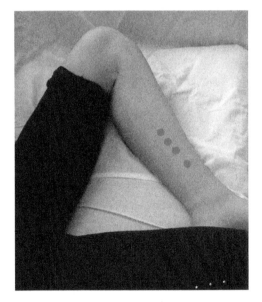

C4   Calf to back

These points on your bladder meridian are on your calves. They are used by acupuncturists for the treatment of lower back, calf and hemorrhoid pain. Your knuckles or massage tools are suitable for massaging them. (See also **L5 Fist to inner calf** on page 132.)

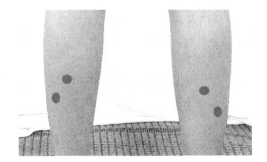

C5   Foot outer edge

Finger pressure is all you will need for these pressure points on the edge of your foot. They are used in acupuncture to strengthen bladder function and sooth lower back and urinary pain.

These pressure points can also be used for ankle sprains.

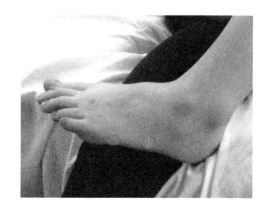

C6   Foot inner edge

These pressure points are used for lower back pain and weakness. When the main arch of the foot collapses, this part of your foot and the opposite knee can get sensitive. Use your knuckle or the Thumbsaver for this. These muscles, though small, can get very stiff and seem to bother people most when the weather is cold.

If you already have a collapsed foot arch, wearing an orthotic shoe insert can help you walk more easily.

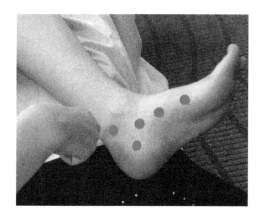

C7   Back of wrist

These acupressure points can relieve wrist and hand pain. These points are also used by acupuncturists to treat lower back and shoulder pain.

Use your fingertips or knuckles to find and press these points between and next to your hand and wrist bones.

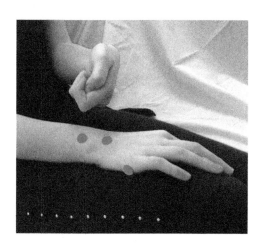

C8   Front of wrist

These acupressure points can be used for carpal tunnel syndrome. They are also used in acupressure and shiatsu to lessen anxiety, nausea and insomnia.

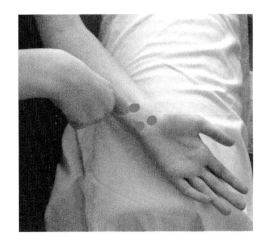

Plastic seasickness prevention bands work by pressing on the dot furthest from the wrist in the photo. Acupuncturists use this point, PC6, for morning sickness too.

C9   Jaw points

These two points on the stomach meridian are easily located: the upper point is just below the cheek bone angle, forward of your ear, and the lower is in the middle of the jaw muscle groove.

Stress, coldness, intense concentration, stimulants, gum chewing and dental problems can all tighten these muscles and cause strong headaches.

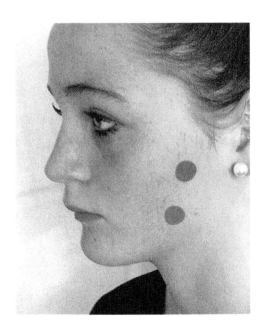

Self Massaging these points can be of assistance to singers and professional speakers for better annunciation. If you have a jaw that clunks when you open and close your mouth, you probably need to regularly massage these points.

Watching someone else's jaw muscles tense is usually a sure sign that they are not happy; it's not as easy to see in oneself.

There have been many times that a client has suddenly told me about their conflict with someone when I massage these points.

C10 Dizzy points

These highlighted points are used a lot by acupuncturists for relieving neck, shoulder and head pain. In TCM (Traditional Chinese Medicine), they are also used for lightheadedness and clumsiness. If any pressure over these points makes your lightheadedness worse, you should desist and see your doctor.

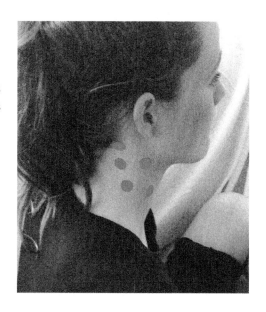

Only press over muscle, not over nor toward your neck arteries or windpipe. In TCM, tinnitus sufferers are treated with some of these pressure points too.

Neck Self Massage techniques **N1 Scalene stroke**, **N2 Scalene stroke with tool**, and **N5 Upward slide** (pages 64 and 66) are all good ways to press these points.

If your lightheadedness results from high or low blood pressure or a middle ear problem, see a doctor.

C11 Back points

There are rows of acupressure points along the thick muscle bands on either side of your spine. Using tennis balls or a foam roller you can slowly rest on each level as you Self Massage. Whether you are standing or lying down, you may be surprised at how sensitive some points are, even under moderate pressure.

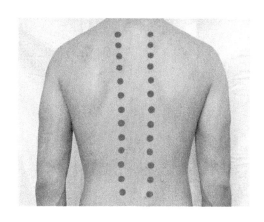

Do this standing before you try it lying down, and use softer balls before you try harder ones.

These points are all located on the bladder meridian and are much used in acupressure, acupuncture and shiatsu. (See also **S5 Two ball wall roll** on page 76 and **X3 Upper back floor balls** on page 154.)

C12 Chest points

These two acupressure points are used to ease breathing and non-heart-related chest muscle pain.

If you have chest pain, get it medically checked out before you try Self Massaging the pain away, especially if you have breathlessness or pain or tingling in your left arm.

The upper point is a couple of inches below the middle of the collarbone and the side point is below the armpit and level with the bottom of the pectoral (chest) muscle. They are often sensitive.

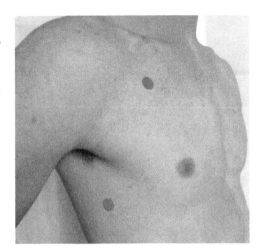

C13 Hip points

This is a group of pressure points that can relieve hip pain and create a greater ease of hip and lower back movement when palpated.

Do not wait for your hip muscles to hurt before you Self Massage them. They will usually be stiff because they are big and strong and get used a lot. They also have few sensory nerve endings, which means they can get really stiff before you even notice them.

These same pressure points can also be used to treat fatigue. Use firmer pressure with these points.

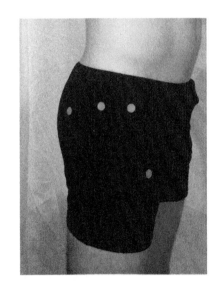

C14 Neck points

These gall bladder meridian points are used extensively in acupressure and shiatsu to bring relief to headaches, neck pain, insomnia, irritability, sore eyes and sinus congestion.

X1 Supine neck ball and **X2 Neck stick** (page 153) can help you Self Massage these points.

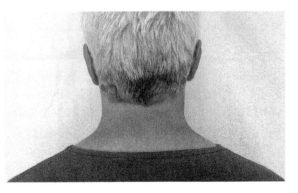

PART IV

Introductory programs for different activities. Golf, a popular 40+ activity, gets its own chapter.

20 PRACTICAL APPLICATIONS

In this chapter, twelve common activities and their associated aches and pains are identified. Examples of Self Massage and exercise are given to improve our ability to do these activities and to lessen the pain and stiffness they can cause.

Each page contains six techniques or exercises. The descriptions are referenced by number and by page. When you go to those pages, you will find other techniques and exercises that work on the same muscles, which you can also try if you like.

Do the Self Massage and exercises as instructed – do not short cut or rush anything. These Self Massage and exercise interventions are there specifically to assist your functional fitness needs.

There are no Advanced Self Massage techniques shown in this chapter because – as always – the easier techniques should be tried first. If you cannot do the easier Self Massage techniques, you will find the Advanced ones way too difficult.

With all Self Massage and exercise, you should stop doing it if it causes pain, nausea or light-headedness.

Golf, a common 40+ activity, has its own chapter starting on page 201.

20.1 CARRYING YOUNG CHILDREN

Even the lightest children can feel increasingly heavy after you have been carrying them for a while. This can really stiffen your upper body, especially when they start to squirm.

Because we like to keep our most useful hand free while we carry our kids and grandkids (so we can open doors, operate microwaves and use the phone, etc.), the load is not shared evenly on both sides of your body.

Typically the muscles on the top of the shoulder and side of the neck on your baby-carrying arm can get very stiff and sore. This is a very common problem for people with young children – a problem that the following Self Massage and exercises can help you manage better.

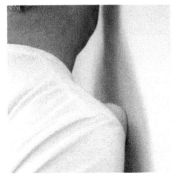
S2 Shoulder wall roll (page 74) loosens the front of your shoulder.

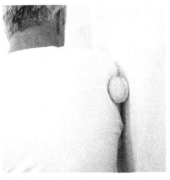
S3 Shoulder blade wall roll (page 75) loosens the back of your shoulder.

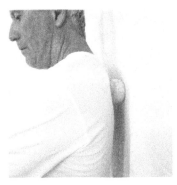
S4 Upper back wall roll (page 75) relieves pain at the top of your shoulder.

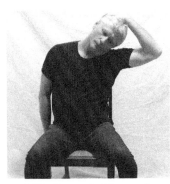
N12 Seated side neck stretch (page 69) stretches the side of your neck.

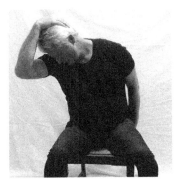
N13 Diagonal neck stretch (page 70) relieves upper shoulder tension.

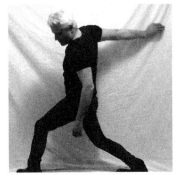
S18 Backward arm stretch (page 83) relieves tension at the front of your shoulder.

20.2 COMPUTER WORK

Even if the ergonomics of your workstation are good, it is very easy to get so absorbed with the task in front of you that you lose awareness of your posture and start to sag in your seat.

The human body is made to move, and some of the most difficult things you can ask of it involve remaining motionless for extended periods of time. Fortunately, there are some useful exercises and Self Massage techniques that you can do in the office environment that can bring some welcome relief to your neck, back and shoulders.

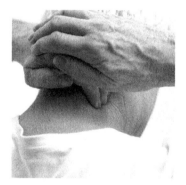

N4 Two hand neck rub (page 65) loosens behind your neck.

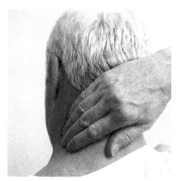

N5 Upward neck slide (page 66) loosens the side and back of your neck.

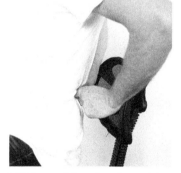

B3 Seated lumbar knuckles (page 115) can be done to relieve back pain without even leaving your seat.

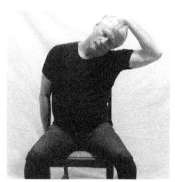

N12 Seated side neck stretch (page 69) stretches the side of your neck.

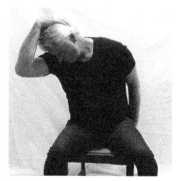

N13 Diagonal neck stretch (page 70) relieves pain and tiredness behind your neck.

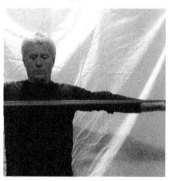

S23 Upper back band flex (page 86) helps to straighten your posture and can be done without leaving your seat.

20.3 GARDENING

Protecting your knees and back are conducive to enjoying your garden. For many of us, gardening is our closest or even our only contact with nature. Bending to weed, using shears and shoveling soil can leave you feeling pretty sore.

Despite the physical difficulty of the work there is a creative satisfaction that gives many retirees hours of enjoyment every week. Seasonal changes keeps it interesting too, a constant reminder of the cycle of life. Whatever your motivation, the following activities can help take the pain out of it.

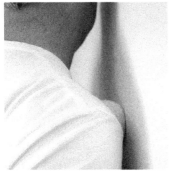

S2 Shoulder wall roll (page 74) relieves stiff gardener's shoulders.

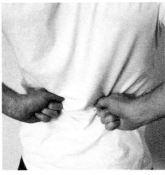

B2 Lumbar knuckles (page 115) can be done standing to relieve lower back pain.

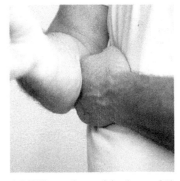

A5 Elbow knuckle (page 97) can ease the tension of repetitious gardening tasks like pruning.

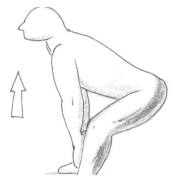

M9 Bending down (page 49) helps you bend down without pain.

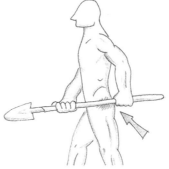

T10 Shovel hip (page 170) is an easy to learn labor saving shoveling technique.

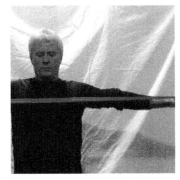

S23 Upper back band flex (page 86) can alleviate some of the more common postural stresses associated with gardening.

20.4 HAIRDRESSING

Hair treatment chemicals, scissor cuts, being on your feet all day, repetitive strain of the hands and working in awkward postures present numerous OH&S problems for hairdressers.

Hairdressing can be a very physically demanding job, and neck and shoulder tension can become particularly intense. If you want to keep doing it, the following Self Massage and exercises can help you.

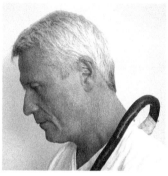

N8 Neck walking stick (page 67) is a good way to de-stress your neck at the end of the day.

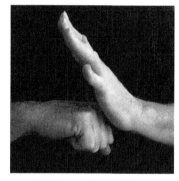

R2 Palm knuckles (page 177) can be done between cuts to loosen your hands.

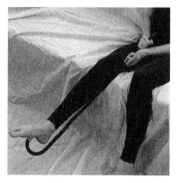

R4 Sole stick press (page 178) sooths your aching feet during your breaks and at the end of the day.

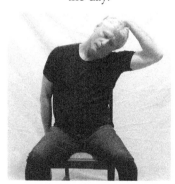

N12 Seated side neck stretch (page 69) must be done on a seat you can hold the side of to relieve neck and shoulder tension.

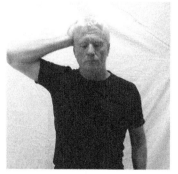

N11 Side neck flex (page 69) can be done sitting or standing to ease and straighten your neck.

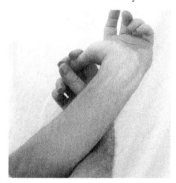

A29 Backward thumb stretch (page 108) relieves hand and thumb tension from scissor use.

20.5 CYCLING

Cycling can be good cardio but it can also distort your posture, strain your shoulders and stiffen your leg muscles. Hamstring and calf muscles shorten the more you ride, because these muscles never fully straighten as you pedal – they get stronger but less flexible.

On a road bike, your back is always bent. Professional cycling teams usually travel with their own therapists partly for this reason. Your shoulders are continually holding your upper body up on road bikes, so road cyclists get sore shoulders. Riding a mountain bike puts you in a better upright posture and is easier on your shoulders (unless you are actually mountain biking on steep tracks).

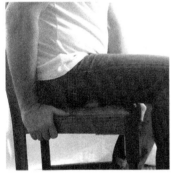

L11 Hamstring ball (page 135) is an easy way to get good controlled massaging pressure into the muscles behind your thigh.

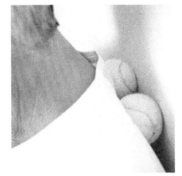

S5 Two ball wall roll (page 76) can relieve both upper back and neck tension.

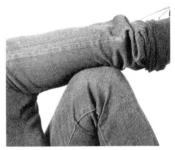

L3 Knee and calf rub (page 131) is an easy relaxing way to loosen your calves after a long ride.

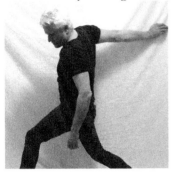

S18 Backward arm stretch (page 83) helps prevent tension and shortening of the muscles at the front of your shoulders and chest.

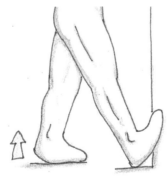

L39 Standing calf stretch (page 145) is a good way to get used to stretching your legs.

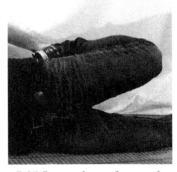

L37 Lateral quad stretch (page 145) helps prevent quad stiffness and shortening. Like your hamstrings, they cannot stretch while you pedal either.

20.6 TENNIS

Tennis can not only give you tennis elbow, but also affect your wrist, lower back and knees. Your elbow and wrist are mainly put under strain by the repeated use of your wrist extensors (muscles on top of the forearm) during backhand strokes.

The sudden changes of direction running on the court can be jarring on the knees. Serving can strain your back as can the lopsided nature of using one arm all the time.

The harder you go, the greater the stress on the joints. But even if you go easy, there is still a problem with keeping even muscle tone on both sides of your body. This has a twisting effect on your posture that should be countered with more even-sided supplementary exercises.

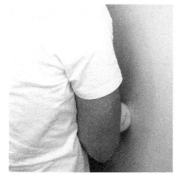

A6 Ball elbow (page 97) is the best Self Massage for your wrist extensors.

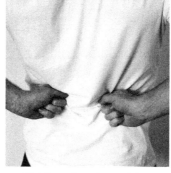

B2 Lumbar knuckles (page 115) is a convenient lower back technique to use while you are on the court.

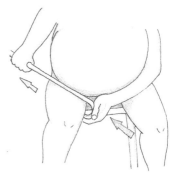

L21 Inner thigh press (page 139) can help loosen stiff thigh muscles and bring relief to knee pain.

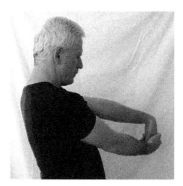

A26 Extensor stretch (page 107) is easy to do anywhere to relieve elbow and wrist tension.

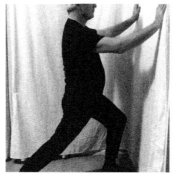

B21 Standing groin stretch (page 124) can help relieve calf, knee and lower back tension.

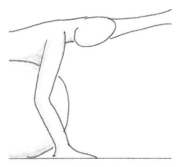

B24 Ball bird dog stretch (page 125) helps straighten your spine, assists coordination and fosters even posture.

20.7 DRIVING

Drivers have similar postural problems to computer workers. Sitting for long periods can give you back pain and is not good for blood circulation in your legs. Unlike computer work, you cannot stand up to give yourself a break whenever you feel like it. Even if you have a good seat, be sure to use it properly (refer to *Posture and driving* on page 22), and take breaks.

Driving for long periods can stiffen your neck, particularly when going long distances staring straight ahead. Long periods of stop/start city and suburban driving can give you stiff calves through constant use of the control pedals.

Delivery drivers are at even more of a disadvantage because they often have to move quickly to discharge their cargo. This can tear muscles that suddenly go from being completely immobile to lifting, carrying and walking fast.

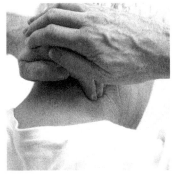

Use **N4 Two hand neck rub** (page 65) while stopped at red lights. Keep your eyes on the road so you are aware of the lights changing.

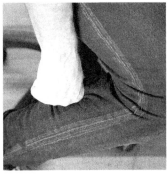

L4 First to outer calf (page 132) can be used while you are stopped too, leaning slightly forward with eyes still on the road.

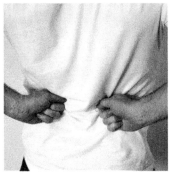

B2 Lumbar knuckles (page 115) can be used when you get out of your vehicle.

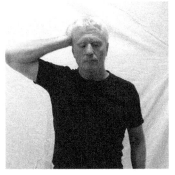

N11 Side neck flex (page 69) can be easily used while stopped at traffic lights.

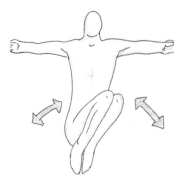

B17 Supine knee rocking (page 122) can be used if your back is particularly sore after driving.

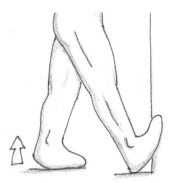

L39 Standing calf stretch (page 145) can be used when you stop and get out of your vehicle.

20.8 POLICE AND SECURITY WORK

Road-based police have to contend with the same postural issues as drivers, with the added burden of a thick duty belt that can weigh over 5 kilograms (10 pounds). Some of the duty belt objects (e.g. torch and baton) can bounce up and down when officers run, which affects balance and movement too.

The equipment on the belt can make sitting awkward and uncomfortable, particularly with the side backrest support that is normally a comfort benefit for drivers and passengers.

Like delivery drivers, police can be suddenly required to run fast from a prolonged sedentary position, which can tear muscles. The same Self Massage and exercise advice applies as for drivers, with extra emphasis on the following.

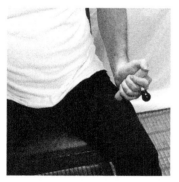

B6 Upper thigh rub (page 117) can be performed while you are waiting for traffic lights to change.

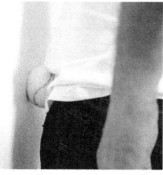

B5 Wall ball hip (page 116) is executed standing against a wall to loosen hip muscles.

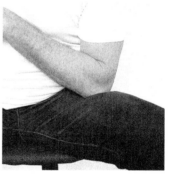

L7 Elbow to thigh (page 116) can loosen your hip muscles too.

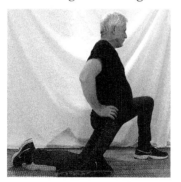

B22 Kneeling groin stretch (page 124) is best used after hip Self Massage. Ease into this stretch.

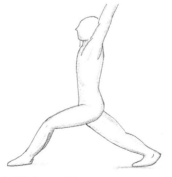

M11 Stretching up (page 50). This Goodman's exercise stretches and strengthens your core simultaneously.

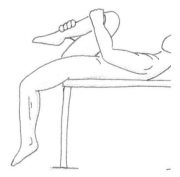

B18 Flexor & butt stretch (page 122) stretches front and back hip muscles at the same time.

195

20.9 MUSICIANS AND ARTISTS

Whether you play wind or string instruments or paint or sculpt, the chances are that you are holding your arms up for extended periods. This can be hard on your shoulders. The angle that the neck is held at can cause pain and stiffness too – violinists are a good example of postural stress at work.

The general body posture of artists and musicians tends to take a poor second place to concentrating on the creation in front of them. Office workers are given OH&S support for their workplace ergonomics, but artists and musicians have to figure things out and police their work practices for themselves.

The more absorbed you are in your headspace, the more the needs of your body get neglected.

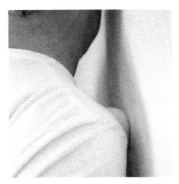

S2 Shoulder wall roll
(page 74) helps loosen chest and shoulder muscles that support your extended arm.

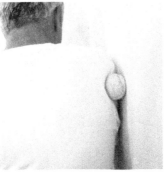

S3 Shoulder blade wall roll
(page 75) relieves shoulder tension from repetitive arm movements.

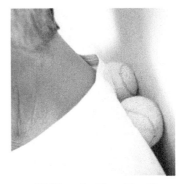

S5 Two ball wall roll
(page 76) can help freshen up tired upper back muscles.

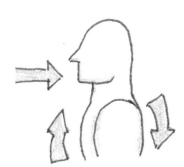

M7 Rolling shoulder stretch (page 48) is an easy stretch to use as you work.

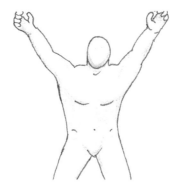

M8 Founder posture
(page 48) is an effective core exercise no matter what the activity is.

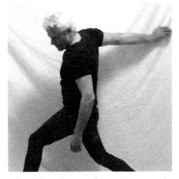

S18 Backward arm stretch
(page 83) opens your chest and shoulders if your arms are held forward for long periods.

20.10 WALKING

Waitresses, hikers, nurses, dog walkers, tour guides and mail deliverers can cover a lot of distance as they work. Even though walking is usually good exercise, we all have our limits of endurance, particularly if we walk fast.

Practical comfortable footwear is required no matter why you are walking. So is paying attention to the ground in front of you.

If you have collapsed foot arches, orthotic shoe inserts can help improve your experience of walking. Be mindful that not all shoe inserts work equally well in all types of shoes.

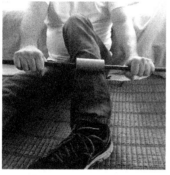

L14 Tibial roll (page 136) can help loosen shin muscle tension.

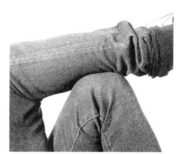

L3 Knee and calf rub (page 131) can be done sitting or lying and is effective in easing stiff calves.

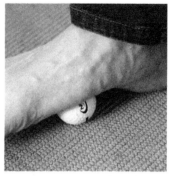

L1 Sole roll (page 131) is a good foot massage. If your feet are very sore, roll a frozen plastic water bottle instead.

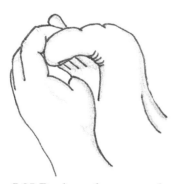

L25 Backward toe stretch (page 141) relieves tension in the ball of your foot.

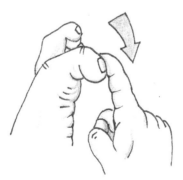

L26 Forward toe stretch (page 48) relieves ankle tension.

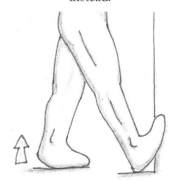

L39 Standing calf stretch (page 145) relieves calf and Achilles tension.

20.11 BACKPACKING

Soldiers, hikers, travellers, school students and mail deliverers carrying medium- to heavy-weight packs are all at risk of lower back injury. You should always make your load even, carry it high on your back and use the chest and waist straps to evenly distribute the load.

Unfortunately, even if you do all these things, the weight could still be too much, especially when carried for too long. Tripping over is more likely to injure you if you carry a big pack and you must be mindful about lifting it into position too.

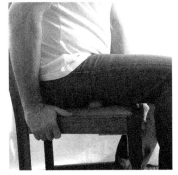

L11 Hamstring ball
(page 135) can relieve leg tension from steep uphill walks.

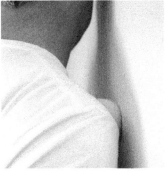

S2 Shoulder wall roll
(page 74) can relieve shoulder tension from pack carrying.

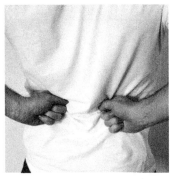

B2 Lumbar knuckles
(page 115) gives lower back tension relief.

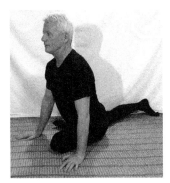

B19 Pigeon stretch
(page 123) stretches the thigh and butt muscles that work hard carrying loads.

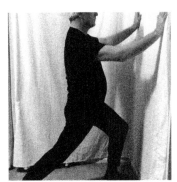

B21 Standing groin stretch
(page 124) relieves hip, calf and thigh tension.

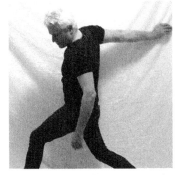

S18 Backward arm stretch
(page 83) helps correct a shoulders-forward posture that can result from backpacking.

20.12 HOUSEWORK

Vacuuming, sweeping and mopping can all produce lower back pain. It is hard keeping good posture when you are in a hurry to do these things. The further you reach forward and sideways, the greater the strain on your back. Move your feet to stay next to the area being cleaned, and change sides to share the workload.

Cleaning tiles, windows and walls can be strenuous on your cleaning arm so share the workload between both hands. It is slower working this way but with practice you can get faster.

If you need to lower your body, move your feet further apart instead of bending your back (see **T4 Giraffe stance** on page 168). Housework is the greatest test of functional fitness.

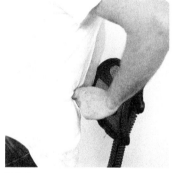

B3 Seated lumbar knuckles (page 115) can relieve back pain from sweeping, vacuuming and mopping.

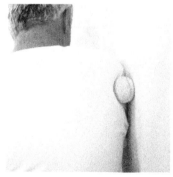

S3 Shoulder blade wall roll (page 75) can relieve shoulder tension from rapid and repetitious cleaning.

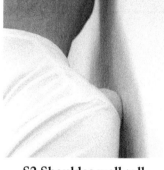

S2 Shoulder wall roll (page 74) helps you keep your shoulders back and down after you finish cleaning.

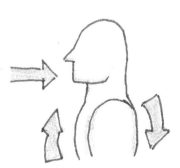

M7 Rolling shoulder stretch (page 48) helps correct upper body posture.

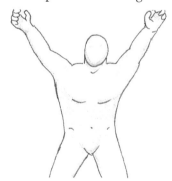

M8 Founder posture (page 48) enhances your upright posture.

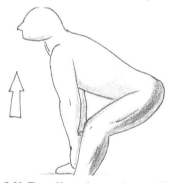

M9 Bending down (page 49) can help get you out of the habit of bending your back when lowering your body.

21 GOLF & YOUR BODY

Golf gets its own chapter because of its popularity with the over-40's – few if any other sports get taken up as much later in life as golf. All sports, including golf, have inherent injury risks, and bodies tend to become more brittle as they age so greater care is needed to prevent injury and maintain normal function. Keeping your joints healthy depends a lot on how you treat your muscles.

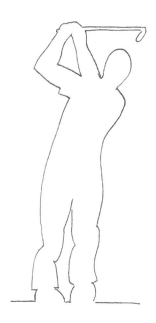

The purpose of this chapter is to help you free your swing, improve your balance and avoid injuries common to golfers, through Self Massage and exercise.

Self Massage techniques are matched with exercise to help you be fit for play. Apart from the walking, golf doesn't really give you much exercise, but exercise can help you play better.

21.1 GOLFER'S HIP AND LOWER BACK

The lower back and hip are not only in close proximity to one another, they are also prone to injury in golfers because of the strong torsion of the most powerful strokes (especially when you hit the ground). As each affects the other, the hip and lower back are discussed together.

By the time most of us turn 40, we have already experienced back or hip pain at least once. There is a fair chance your lower back or hips are not in pristine condition before the first stroke is even played.

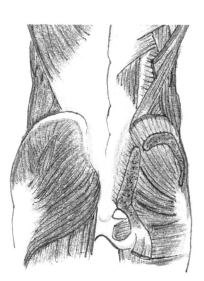

Lower back and hip strain are less likely if your back is strong and flexible. Strength and flexibility are both required to properly enjoy your play.

It is best practice is to get some professional massage before you start tearing up the course. The massage therapist can advise you where to apply Self Massage. Take this book with you and they can show you what Self Massage techniques and exercises you should do.

Get golfing lessons from a professional before you play.

The following Self Massage techniques can all give you relief of lower back stiffness and discomfort. They can also help make lower back exercises easier to perform. You can do these Self Massage techniques while you are out on the course between holes.

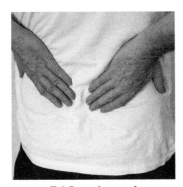

B1 Lumbar rub
(page 115)

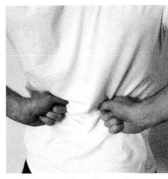

B2 Lumbar knuckles
(page 115)

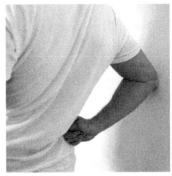

B4 Lumbar wall lean
(page 116)

Goodman's Foundation Training exercises on pages 47 to 50 are good for your back too. Like the back Self Massage above, they can be done indoors or outdoors, require no equipment and can be done standing up. These are exercises you can do on the course. 30 to 60 seconds is plenty of time to do one or more of these exercises between strokes.

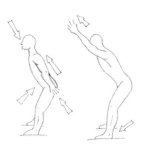
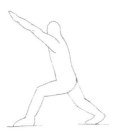
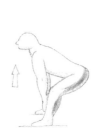
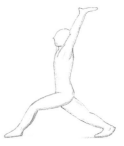

The following exercises and Self Massage techniques can help you be golf fit too, but are not nearly as practical to use on the course. If you find getting down onto the floor and getting up again difficult, try doing them on a firm bed. Instructions on how to perform these exercises can be found on the referenced pages.

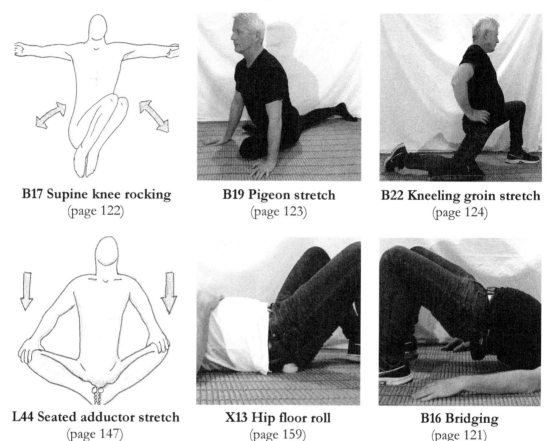

B17 Supine knee rocking
(page 122)

B19 Pigeon stretch
(page 123)

B22 Kneeling groin stretch
(page 124)

L44 Seated adductor stretch
(page 147)

X13 Hip floor roll
(page 159)

B16 Bridging
(page 121)

G1   MIT hip strengthening exercise

MIT devised this strengthening exercise specifically for golfers' hip ligaments. If you have not tried this before, hold something stable for support. Your balance can benefit from doing this too. Aim to do 20 seconds on each side. If you get dizziness or pain, stop at once.

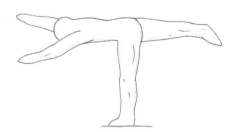

Your supporting leg should be straight, with your other leg and arms outstretched and level. If you manage to master this with your eyes open, try it with your eyes closed too.

21.2 GOLFER'S KNEE

Your knees are prone to movements while playing golf that can be stressful to ligaments and cartilage. The sudden sideways shifting of body weight inside the joint capsule during approach shots can stir up old injuries, as well as cause new ones. Added to this is the cartilage thinning that occurs with the normal aging process.

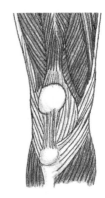

Golf Digest recommends the leg exercises starting on page 205 to help prevent golf-related knee injuries. If you practice the following Self Massage techniques first, the exercises will be easier to do. The walking stick Self Massage techniques in Chapter 14 can be useful for Golfer's knee too. Most of us have stiff legs, and playing golf well is just one of the things stiff knees stop us from doing.

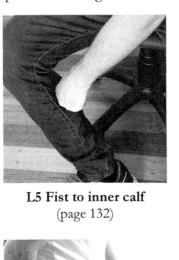

L5 Fist to inner calf
(page 132)

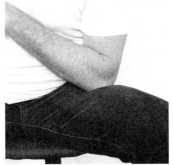

L7 Elbow to thigh
(page 133)

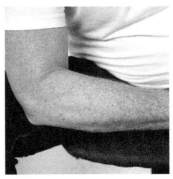

L8 Adductor press
(page 134)

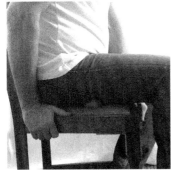

L11 Hamstring ball
(page 135)

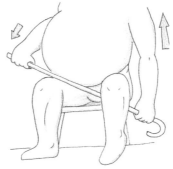

L22 Hamstring stick
(page 140)

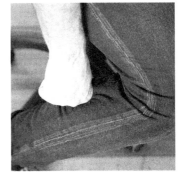

L4 First to outer calf
(page 132)

Do not Self Massage over varicose veins. If you get pain in your calf that does not respond well to exercise or massage, see your doctor, as it may be a DVT or compartment syndrome.

The following exercises are recommended by Golf Digest to help strengthen your knees. If you are short or have very stiff legs, use a lower chair.

G2 Step and reach

Place one foot on a chair with the other out behind you and reach straight up, pushing your hips forward as you do so.

Hold for 20 seconds and then do the other side. Remember to push your hips forward as you reach upward.

If the leading knee is sore doing this, try moving the foot on the floor slightly back so the forward knee is not bent as acutely.

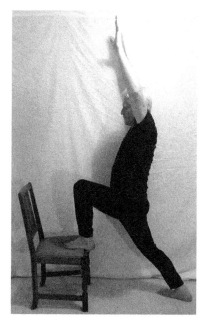

G3 Chair pushdown

This is a thigh strengthening exercise. With one foot forward and the other pressing down against a chair behind you, hold this position until the muscle **starts** to tire. This may take only a few seconds to start with, so gradually extend the time with regular practice.

Like all other exercises that require balancing on one leg, be close enough to something stable so you can steady yourself against it if needed.

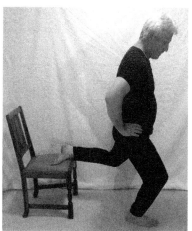

The following stretching exercises are recommended by Golf Digest. It is important to adopt the right posture with these stretches or they won't work properly. Do these exercises between playing, rather than as a warm-up. Brisk walking and percussive massage are more useful for warm-up.

G4 Chair stretch

With one foot forward and the other stretched back, hold a chair as shown to give you support for balance. If the knee in your backward stretched leg feels too pressured against the floor, place a cushion beneath it or use stretch **B21 Standing groin stretch** (page 124) instead. Hold for at least 20 seconds and then do the other side.

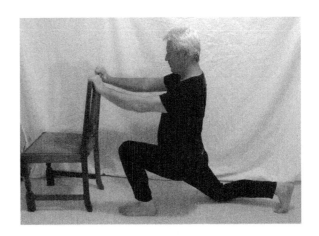

Hip flexor and quad stretches like this lessen the tension in both the hip and knee joints.

G5 Hamstring chair

Stand with one leg straightened out in front of you with your heel pushing downward onto the chair in front of you. This exercise has a side benefit of improving your balance by engaging the muscles in the sole of the foot you are standing on. Hold for 20 seconds and then do the other side.

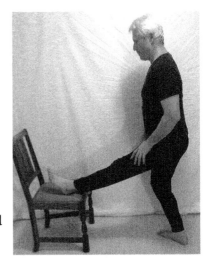

If this is hard to do with a chair, place your foot on something lower such as a step or a foot stool.

If you find it too difficult to balance and stretch at the same time (with toes pointed up), do stretch **L38 Seated hamstring stretch** (page 145) instead.

At the time of writing this book, research was in the process of creating artificial knee replacements better suited to the rigors of playing golf than existing knee joint replacements. Existing artificial knees are even less suited to the rigors of sideways weight shifting than normal knees are.

So if you are a keen golfer with knees beyond help, there is hope on the horizon.

21.3 GOLFER'S ELBOW

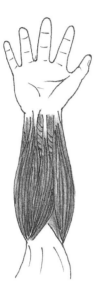

Golfer's elbow (medial epicondylitis) is a repetitive strain injury that causes pain and stiffness on the inner side of the elbow joint. The lower hand on the club (the right hand on a right-handed golfer and the left hand on a left-hander) snaps forward at the wrist in order to flight the ball.

Press your thumb over the muscle just below your elbow on the inner side of your forearm and move your wrist back and forth. Can you feel the muscle flex as you cock your wrist forward? Golfer's elbow is a condition that amateurs are statistically more likely to get than professionals because of the wrist action of playing chip shots out of bunkers and long grass. The more shots you play out of the rough, the worse it gets.

Many golfers get some relief from strapping the elbow with a band around the arm just below the elbow, but for even better results, try the following Self Massage and exercises.

A5 Elbow knuckle (page 97)

This is a good Self Massage technique to bring relief to golfer's elbow. Place your fist against your lower rib cage and move the inner side of the forearm back and forth over your knuckles. The fist stays still against your ribs. If the elbow is already inflamed, only work as close to the joint as comfort will allow. This is an easy Self Massage to use on the course between strokes.

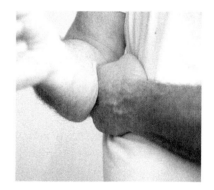

G6   Wall press

This is applied by knuckle pressure with the back of your forearm against the wall. Work from the wrist toward the elbow.

Softening the muscle first with Self Massage can make the stretches on the next page more comfortable and effective. Do not apply pressure directly over the boney part of your elbow.

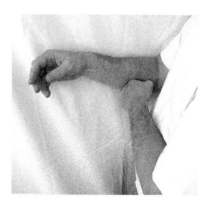

The stiff muscles that produce hyperextension and hyperflexion strains require stretching more than strengthening exercises. The following stretching exercises will help, and are easy stretches to do almost anywhere. Any task that requires the frequent grasping of objects can also tighten these busy muscles. Hold each stretch for a minimum of 20 seconds. Stretch each finger backward in **A28** for 20 seconds.

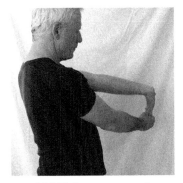

A24 Palm up stretch
(page 106)

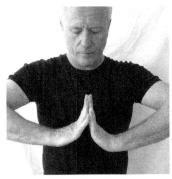

A25 Prayer stretch
(page 106)

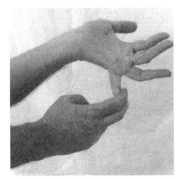

A28 Backward finger stretch
(page 108)

21.4 Golfer's wrist

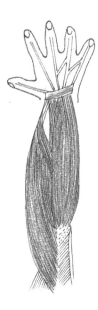

Golfer's wrist is caused by wrist hyperextension and repetitive strain of the wrist extensors. Approach shots cause it. When your leading wrist flexes backward and compresses the back of the joint, this can create a pinching sensation that leads to pain and inflammation. As with golfer's elbow, you are more likely to get it if you play out of the rough a lot.

This injury is usually referred to as tennis elbow (lateral epicondylitis) because it is common in tennis players. You can get tennis elbow even though you may never have picked up a tennis racquet. Because golfer's wrist and tennis elbow are basically caused by the same action, the Self Massage and exercises for both are the same.

Apart from playing golf and tennis, your wrist extensors can be strained by repeatedly picking up things with an overhand grip like bricklayers do or from zip-starting mowers and chainsaws often. Sufferers of golfer's wrist can experience a weakening of grip. Ice packs can relieve the acute symptoms, as can Self Massage and stretching.

The following Self Massage and stretching techniques help golfer's wrist and tennis elbow. In the stretches, your wrist extensors are stretched as your wrist is passively flexed forward. Hold each stretch for 20 seconds and then do the other side.

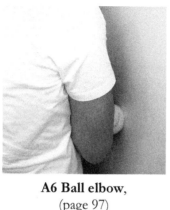

A6 Ball elbow,
(page 97)

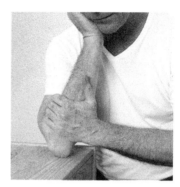

A7 Elbow ratchet rub
(page 98)

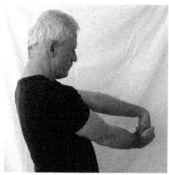

A26 Extensor stretch
(page 107)

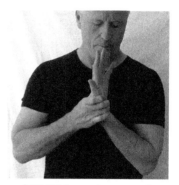

A27 Wrist twist stretch
(page 107)

21.5 GOLFER'S SHOULDER

Golfer's shoulders are subject to hyperextension strains due to the high back lift and follow through of the swing. Shoulders are not naturally strong when your hands are strenuously engaged in activities above shoulder height or behind the center line of your body. 30% of the total golf swing is in that zone.

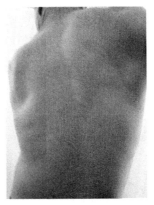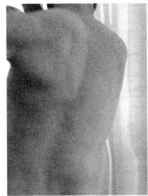

Learning how to swing properly from a pro can save you much suffering later on. Trying to belt the spots off the ball with bad playing posture and stiff shoulder muscles can damage your rotator cuff, which can necessitate surgery.

Look at the above photos of the backswing (left) and the follow through (right). Those muscles you can see working so hard do so better when regularly Self Massaged and stretched. Feel the muscles in your chest and the front of your shoulder in turn with one hand while slowly swinging the other arm back and forth in front of yourself. Self Massaging and stretching those same muscles will help free your swing too.

Golf – like the racquet and bat-and-ball sports – needs to be countered with even-postured exercises. Chin-ups and push-ups are examples of upper body exercises that can help even up your right and left shoulder strength.

It won't take you long to figure out which shoulder is stiffest at the front and which shoulder feels worse at the back. The following Self Massage techniques are useful for golfers. Start with a softer ball – it is important to be able to relax into the pressure. This should feel good, not painful.

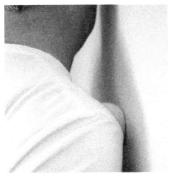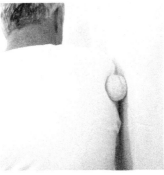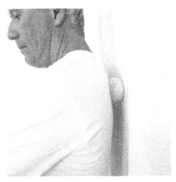

S2 Shoulder wall roll
(page 74)

S3 Shoulder blade wall roll
(page 75)

S4 Upper back wall roll
(page 75)

After the muscles feel looser, they will respond better to stretching. The following stretches will stretch all the muscles in your shoulder that you use for golf. Smoothly ease yourself into each of them. Don't bounce at the end of any stretch, but use a smooth gradual motion from start to finish.

Please follow the exercise descriptions given on the referenced pages.

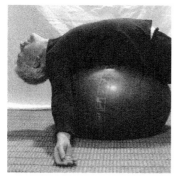
S19 Backward ball stretch
(page 84)

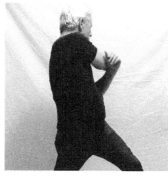
S25 Rotated body stretch
(page 87)

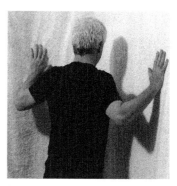
S20 Corner shoulder stretch
(page 85)

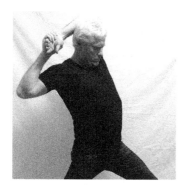
A12 Backward triceps stretch
(page 100)

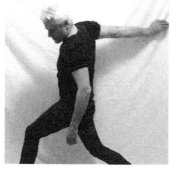
S18 Backward arm stretch
(page 83)

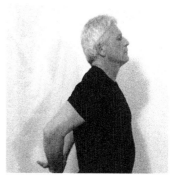
S21 Open chest stretch
(page 85)

21.6 GOLFER'S NECK

Golfers are always turning their heads in the same direction when playing a stroke. Not nearly with the same torsion as in the shoulders or lower back, but enough to create an uneven neck posture that can lead to pain and stiffness or headaches.

Because of its proximity to the shoulders, the neck often suffers when your stroke is particularly forceful and uncontrolled. The neck and shoulder are related, like the hip and lower back.

You may be unaware of the degree to which windy weather can affect the way your neck feels. As an experiment, wear a lightweight scarf around your neck the next time you go to the course. If your neck feels warm and comfortable, your posture and swing can improve as a result.

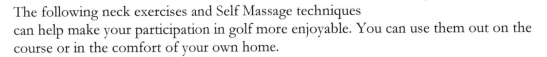

The following neck exercises and Self Massage techniques can help make your participation in golf more enjoyable. You can use them out on the course or in the comfort of your own home.

After your neck is massaged, it will usually stretch better and feel more comfortable. If your general posture is poor off the course, it will probably require some attention on the course.

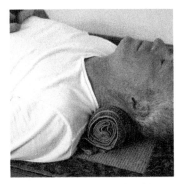

N3 Neck towel roll
(page 65)

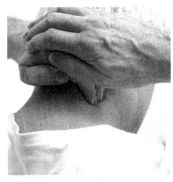

N4 Two hand neck rub
(page 65)

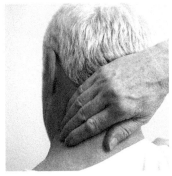

N5 Upward neck slide
(page 66)

The following neck exercises not only contribute to better spinal posture, they can also make your neck feel more comfortable. They can be done sitting or standing. Hold each for at least 20 seconds and then do the other side.

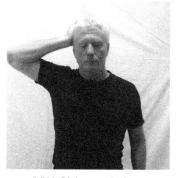

N11 Side neck flex
(page 69)

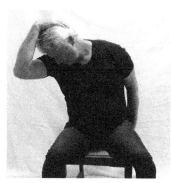

N13 Diagonal neck stretch
(page 70)

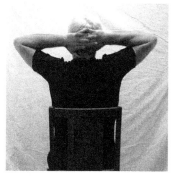

N14 Back of neck flex
(page 70)

If any of these exercises gives you nausea, dizziness or pain, stop. They should feel good, not bad.

21.7 GOLF WARM-UP

Percussive Self Massage is a commonly seen warm-up before tai chi classes and is used by athletes in the Chinese track and field team in their warm-ups too. Percussive Self Massage has a stimulating effect on the nervous system, rather than the sedating affect of the slower and more steady-pressured Self Massage techniques.

If you follow the instructions in the Percussive Self Massage chapter, you will be able to evaluate its worth as a warm-up method for yourself. Remember to let your wrists flap loosely as you strike your muscles with your hands.

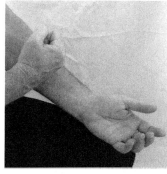

P1 Arm pound
(page 163)

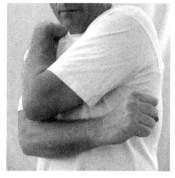

P2 Side pound
(page 163)

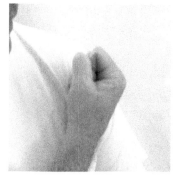

P8 Chest pound
(page 165)

P1, **P2** and **P8** are good examples of Percussive Self Massage techniques that can give your body an invigorating warm-up before a round of golf. All 10 techniques in the Percussive Self Massage chapter can be used in a golf warm-up for your arms, legs and body.

Stretching exercise is no longer recommended as a warm-up routine, as recent studies have shown there is no benefit to performance and it can even lead to injury.

Other exercises like rolling your arms around as you briskly walk will warm your body up quickly. Warm muscles do not tear as easily as cold muscles. There is no reason why neuromotor exercises cannot be used for a golf warm-up either. A few minutes of tai chi can help your balance, which is useful if you want to play up to your potential.

Modern professional golfers are much fitter and well-massaged than they have been in the past. They do this because it helps them play better and for longer. If you regularly approach your game the same way, you should play better and for longer too.

21.8 MATCHING NEEDS TO OUTCOMES

Golf is only one example of how Self Massage and exercise can be combined to produce physical benefits suited to your needs.

Any sport played long enough and hard enough will produce wear and tear on your body. If you want to avoid injury, whether it is through trauma or repetitive strain, Self Massage and exercise can help you.

Golf was chosen not only because it is a sport popular with my target reader demographic but also because golf can play havoc with your muscles and joints. I have treated many golfers over the years. Look closely at the postures and movements that golf is played with and you can see numerous stress loadings that can injure joints.

Good technique unquestionably helps you not only play better but avoid injury too. Self Massage and appropriate exercise assists your technique because it helps your joints achieve and maintain normal comfortable movement.

It is best to be proactive rather than reactive – if you wait until you start to stiffen up, you are more likely to need physiotherapy, therapeutic massage or chiropractic treatment to get playing again. If you do regular Self Massage and exercise you are less likely to stiffen up. Remember that "an ounce of prevention is better than a pound of cure."

No matter what your game, job or hobby, make it more enjoyable for yourself and do it with a comfortable body. If you get joint or muscle pain, look for the Self Massage techniques and exercises that match the location of your pain or stiffness. **However, if your attempts at helping yourself just seem to make you feel worse, see a health professional.**

FURTHER READING

BOOKS

Kaptchuk, Ted, *The Web That Has No Weaver: Understanding Chinese Medicine*
Rider Health Books, 1983
ISBN 0-7126-1172-X

This popular book is a good introduction to the principles of Chinese medicine. It explains the health nexus between mind and body from an oriental holistic tradition.

Greene, Lauriann, *Save Your Hands! Injury Prevention for Massage Therapists*
Gilded Age Press, 1995
ISBN 0-9679549-0-8

Although this book has not been written for Self Massage, the observations made in it about protecting your hands and body from work-related RSI and postural stress are quite astute.

Masunaga & Ohashi, *Zen Shiatsu*
Japan Publications, 1977
ISBN 0-87040-394-x

If the Self Acupressure & Shiatsu chapter was of interest to you, this book can enlighten you about the principles behind it, such as the role of breathing during massage and meridian theory.

WEBSITES

Berube, Jennifer, *Working Ergonomics: The backbone of office ergonomics*
http://workingergonomics.wordpress.com

This website gives good advice on how to avoid repetitive strain injuries and postural problems with sedentary office jobs. Some good ergonomic office furniture is showcased with practical strategies for protecting your back and joints.

Goodman, Eric, *Foundation Training: From pain to performance*
http://www.foundationtraining.com/

I highly recommend this website. It contains effective and practical instruction on core exercises that can improve your postural and neuromotor fitness. Goodman is a chiropractor who has developed an exercise regime based on yoga that strengthens core muscles.

Lieberman, Daniel MD, *Running bare foot*

http://barefootrunning.fas.harvard.edu

This website gives some persuasive advice on the virtues of running barefoot, particularly on grass tracks. Lieberman states that running this way is not only less abrasive to the foot and joints, but also has advantages for your speed, balance and agility.

Fiore, Don, *Qigong videos*

https://www.youtube.com/user/taichihealthproducts/search?query=qigong+tai+chi

Don Fiore has a series of short and easy to follow tai chi and qigong videos that serve as a good introduction to these ancient neuromotor exercise systems. The styles that Fiore demonstrates are quite accessible for older people with no previous experience.

Mandal AC, MD, *Balanced sitting posture on a forward sloping seat*

http://acmandal.com

Dr. Mandal cites research from orthopedic surgeon Dr. J. J. Keegan, who linked sitting for long periods with lower back pain and spinal degeneration (1953). Dr. Keegan used X-ray analysis to determine that the best seating to use is one that opens your hip joint out to a 135-degree angle, as seen with saddle seating.

ARTICLES

Field T (2005),
Cortisol decreases & Serotonin& Dopamine increases following massage
http://www.tandfonline.com/doi/full/10.1080/00207450590956459

This is a health research abstract summarizing findings on the effects of massage on mood-altering hormones. If you are interested in health research and like to see the evidence, it is an informative article about how massage can help stress-related problems.

Goodyer, Paula, *A dose of strong medicine* (2006)
http://www.smh.com.au/news/fitness/a-dose-of-strong-medicine/2006/07/12/1152637736876.html

This is a newspaper article published about a weight training trial for middle-aged and elderly people who experienced strength, muscle mass and general well-being benefits after a six-week trial at a Sydney hospital. Its oldest participant was a 102-year-old woman.

LIST OF TECHNIQUES & EXERCISES

FUNCTIONAL FITNESS

NECK & JAW

Upper Body

ARMS & HANDS

Lower Body

Legs & Feet

Advanced Self Massage

Percussive Self Massage

PRACTICAL POSTURAL TIPS

SELF MASSAGE & REFLEXOLOGY

Self Acupressure & Shiatsu

Golf & Your Body

INDEX

CPSIA information can be obtained
at www.ICGtesting.com
Printed in the USA
BVOW10s0808170416

4022BVAU00005B/1/P